SOAP MAKING FOR BEGINNERS

How to Make Homemade Soap Bars for Beginners

(Different Types of Soap Making With Pictures Illustrations)

Michael Molloy

Published by Oliver Leish

Michael Molloy

All Rights Reserved

Soap Making for Beginners: How to Make Homemade Soap Bars for Beginners (Different Types of Soap Making With Pictures Illustrations)

ISBN 978-1-77485-079-4

Legal & Disclaimer

suggested remedies, techniques, or information in this book.

Upon using the information contained in this book, you agree to hold harmless the Author from and against any damages, costs, and expenses, including any legal fees potentially resulting from the application of any of the information provided by this guide. This disclaimer applies to any damages or injury caused by the use and application, whether directly or indirectly, of any advice or information presented, whether for breach of contract, tort, negligence, personal injury, criminal intent, or under any other cause of action.

You agree to accept all risks of using the information presented inside this book. You need to consult a professional medical practitioner in order to ensure you are both able and healthy enough to participate in this program.

Table of Contents

Introduction

A big hello and welcome, would-be soap wizards. The very fact that you are considering this book already means that you are a pretty crafty person and are either looking for a whole new set of skills or to take your current skill set to the next level.

Soap crafting is a really fun hobby to get into and is easy to learn. It also never gets boring – once you understand the basics of how to create your perfect soaps, you can mix and match ingredients, adding colors and scents or switching molds to create something new every single time.

Whether you are aiming to learn how to make soaps just to pass the time or if you want to make personalized gifts or even turn a profit, soap crafting can provide the answer for you.

Whatever your reason, say goodbye to last-minute trips to the mall to get presents for people – you will have your own on tap supply.

And once you have been bitten by the bug, it will be impossible to go back. I have not bought a commercially-produced bar of soap in decades and my skin has simply never been healthier.

The best way to describe the difference between home-made soap and commercially produced soap is to consider the difference between fresh farm butter and margarine. Both with do the job they are meant to but the butter is so much richer and luxurious and, as it turns out, far better for your health.

If you are looking for an alternative to harsh chemicals and synthetic additives, this book is for you. If you want to make real soap – soap that is both gentle and cleansing, this book is for you.

In this book, we will go through the basics when it comes to cold-process soap crafting. We will deal with how the process works, what ingredients you will need and what quantities of each to use. We will give you a detailed safety list and a full list of equipment necessary. Because this is a book on natural soap crafting, we will steer clear of synthetic fragrances and colorants relying on natural alternatives. We will also go through making your own clear glycerin soap – a lot of fun and a very different process than what you are currently used to.

We end the book with a chapter about common problems and how you can solve them and then a cheat sheet with the main information summarized on it for you to refer to later on.

 So how about it? Are you ready to dive in and start making your own soap? Thought so, let's go!

Chapter 1: Soap Making 101

Soap making is an age-old tradition, which has almost vanished due to the availability of commercial soaps. While people from yesteryears didn't have a choice but to make their own soap, more people these days are opting for handmade soaps as a natural alternative to chemical-rich, store-bought soaps.

But how is soap exactly made?

What most people don't know about soap is that it's actually salt. If you still remember your high school chemistry, you'll know that salt is a product of the chemical reaction between an acid and a base. Indeed, soap is made from an animal- or plant-derived fats and oils (which are acids) and lye (which is a base).

When these two are combined, a chemical reaction known as saponification takes place. But soap isn't the only product of this reaction. During saponification, glycerin—a chemical compound that moisturizes the skin—is formed as a natural byproduct.

Lye is a dangerous chemical because of its high alkalinity. One drop can burn the skin or cause permanent eye damage if not rinsed properly. It's the potential danger of lye and the seemingly intimidating process that keep many people from soap making.

Fortunately for you, you can now make your own handmade soap with or without lye. The methods that involve lye and those that don't are entirely different. But whichever method you choose, you'll find that soap making is fun and fulfilling.

Choosing Essential Equipment and Ingredients

Before you can start making soap, you need to have the necessary materials. You don't need high-end apparatus but you need to gather equipment and ingredients that are suitable for soap making. Below is a list of the must-haves and what to consider when purchasing them.

Soap Making Equipment

Digital Scale

In soap making, all the oils, butters, water, and lye must be measured by weight and not by volume. This is because measuring cups from different manufacturers can vary in size. There's also the tendency of anyone who uses these cups to fill them with less or more. Although the difference may be small, you could end up with a soap that's too oily or lye-heavy, which is unsafe.

You don't need a fancy scale when making soap. You can get one from any store selling kitchen supplies.

Containers

You need several containers:

For measuring lye

Use small disposable cups or a small container marked with the word lye.

For mixing lye

When you add to water, the solution can heat up to 200°F so it's important to use a heat-proof container. A heavy-duty plastic container with a recycle #5 symbol or a stainless steel container is best. Avoid using glass since reaction with lye can cause weak points and accidental breakage.

For measuring/holding liquid oil

You can use any type of container since this will only hold the liquid oils before you add them to the melted solid oils.

For melting oils/soap base and mixing soap

Depending on how you will melt the oils, you can use a microwave-safe bowl, Pyrex mixing pitcher, or a large pot. This container should be big enough to mix all the ingredients and deep enough so you can mix the batter without splashing it around.

For mixing different color

Some recipes may require you to divide the soap batter so you can color them separately. You can use any container except for aluminum or anything with Teflon since they react negatively to the soap batter.

Thermometer

When working with lye, you'll have to add or mix ingredients within a certain temperature range. To do this, you should have a reliable and accurate thermometer.

You can use a candy thermometer if that's what you already have. But for ease of use and convenience, it's best to invest in an infrared thermometer. This tool can tell you the temperature in less than a second with high accuracy. And because it doesn't use a probe, there's no need to clean it after each use.

Stick Blender (Immersion Blender)

Soap making involves a lot of mixing and stirring. Even though you can definitely mix soap by hand, it's time-consuming and could take hours depending on the ingredients and how much soap you're making. With a stick or immersion blender, you can cut that time to just a few minutes.

When you're just starting, it's fine to use an inexpensive stick blender. But if you intend to make soap regularly, it's wise to have a durable blender.

Spoons and Spatulas

You will use these for preparing the lye solution, stirring the oils and soap batter, and scraping bits of soap left in the mixing pot. Choose spoons or spatulas made with silicone or heavy-duty plastic, and go for those with long handles. Avoid anything with aluminum.

Safety Gears

Gloves and goggles are an absolute must when you're working with lye. This chemical is caustic and can leave burn marks on your skin.

Use dishwashing or disposable nitrile or latex gloves to protect your hands. To protect your eyes, use safety goggles specifically made for handling chemicals.

Soap Molds

There are so many types and shapes of molds you can use when making soap. They range from pricey wooden molds to free repurposed containers and boxes.

Silicone Molds

Molds made with silicone are the best because they're ready to use as is and they come in different shapes and sizes. They're quite flexible so they make the removal of soap a breeze. If you're using a mold with individual cavities, there's no need to cut the soap.

When using silicone molds, you have to insulate them well if you want your cold-process soap to fully gel.

Wooden loaf and slab molds

Soap in wooden mold normally doesn't require added insulation to gel, unless it's cold. If you're going to use this type of mold, you have to line it with wax paper or freezer paper. It's also best to choose a mold that's made with untreated hardwood since unsaponified soap can react to treated wood.

PVC pipes

These are great for making round soap. You don't have to line them but smearing some mineral oil will help make the removal of soap much easier.

Plastic or cardboard food *containers*

Yogurt cups, milk cartons, and cream cheese containers can be used as molds. These are great if you're just starting out, you're working with small batches, or there's leftover soap after you've poured into your prepared mold. They don't have to be lined and once soap hardens, you can simply peel the container away.

Tupperware containers/plastic boxes

You don't need to line these molds unless they're thick and not that flexible. Soap should be insulated well to achieve a full gel.

Cardboard boxes

Cardboard boxes, such as sturdy shoe boxes, need to be lined when used as molds. Proper insulation is also necessary for this one.

Cutting Board and Knife/Soap Cutter

If you're making melt-and-pour soap, you'll have to cut the soap base, which comes in large blocks, so they'll melt faster. And if you put your soap in a large mold, you'll have to cut it when it becomes firm.

Other supplies

Spray bottle of alcohol – to remove bubbles and make layers of soap stick together, if you're making melt-and-pour soap; to reduce the formation of soda ash

Paper towels and white vinegar – to wipe away and neutralize spills of lye or splashes of raw soap

Small bowls – for measuring and holding essential oil, fragrance oil, colorants, and other additives

Wax paper – for lining or covering molds

Cardboard and towel/blanket – to cover and insulate the soap

Soap Making Ingredients

Oils, Fats, and Butters

Most soap recipes contain 3 to 6 oils and kinds of butter. Different oils contribute to different properties and knowing these will give you an idea what to expect with your soap in terms of hardness, conditioning, lather, and creaminess.

Apricot kernel oil is high in vitamins A, C, and E. It's highly conditioning, moisturizing, and absorbs easily. It produces a stable creamy lather with small bubbles. This oil is lightweight and using too much (more than 15%) will make soap bars that are too soft and won't last long in the shower.

Argan oil makes soap feel silky. It's highly moisturizing, as well as rich in antioxidants and vitamins A and E.

Avocado butter has a creamy consistency. It moisturizes the skin and makes it feel smooth.

Avocado oil is high in amino acids, beta-carotene, potassium, protein, and vitamins A, B, D, and E. It helps in healing sun-damaged skin and is good for mature or aging skin. Avocado oil in soaps makes it soft so your soap should only have up to 20% of it.

Babassu oil comes from a certain type of palm tree. It's high in antioxidants and vitamin E, and good for both oily and dry skin. Because of its cleansing and firming properties, it can replace palm or coconut oil in a cold-process soap recipe.

Beeswax will add a bit of hardness to your soap and is a great addition to shampoo bars. It's only used in small amounts in soap making since it reduces lather. It also speeds up trace so if it's your first time making cold-process soap, avoid those recipes that include beeswax.

Black cumin seed oil or black seed oil has anti-oxidants and anti-inflammatory properties. It's known as a natural skincare and haircare aid. It can be used to make a gentle cleanser that soothes irritated skin.

Canola oil gives the soap a dense creamy lather. It's inexpensive and can be used as an alternative for olive oil.

Castor oil is a thick liquid derived from the castor bean plant. It is easily absorbed into the skin and creates a soap with amazing lather. It's great for making shampoo bars, too. Ideally, your soap shouldn't have more than 10% of castor oil since too much can make it soft and sticky.

Cocoa butter makes soap extra moisturizing and feels luxurious. It should only be used in small amounts since too much may cause soap to crack or easily melt.

Coconut oil is one of the most common oils used in soap making and it's known for its excellent cleansing power. However, it strips oils off the skin as it cleanses so if you're making soap for dry or sensitive skin, make sure that it doesn't have more than 15% of coconut oil.

Flaxseed oil contains essential fatty acids in the right proportion that gives it special healing and skin-renewing properties. You can use up to 5% of this oil in cold-process soap.

Grapeseed oil is lightweight, thin, and high in antioxidants. It's non-comedogenic, making it great for oily or acne-prone skin. Soaps with this oil can make your skin feel silky smooth.

Hazelnut oil moisturizes while cleansing the skin and is suitable for all skin types.

Hemp seed oil contains many nutrients and is rich in fatty acids. It helps keep skin hydrated and is great for dry or aging skin. Soaps with hemp seed oil make excellent lather but they also have a relatively shorter shelf life.

Jojoba oil is more like liquid wax. It contributes to a long-lasting bar of soap. It should only be used in small amounts since too much may weigh down the lather and cause pores to clog.

Lard is fat derived from pork. Recipes using lard are great for beginners since it's cheap. It also makes a long-lasting bar with a creamy lather. Freshly made soap with lard can smell like bacon but this goes away after curing.

Mango butter is high in antioxidants and vitamins A and E. It's semi-solid, melting once it touches the skin. It contributes to the soap's hardness and creates a stable, conditioning lather. Mango butter is good for dry and aging skin.

Olive oil is a thick oil that is known for its excellent moisturizing power. It's high in antioxidants but has little cleansing property. Olive oil is mild enough to be used for sensitive skin. It's great for all skin types, including a baby's skin. Pure olive oil makes a soft soap so it's best combined with hard oils or fat. Never use extra-virgin olive oil in soap making.

Palm kernel oil produces a hard cleansing bar with long-lasting lather. It can speed up trace, so only work with recipes using palm kernel oil when you're already confident with your soap-making skills. It's possible to replace this oil in a recipe with babassu or coconut oil.

Palm oil produces a hard, long-lasting bar of soap with creamy lather when combined with coconut oil. This oil is controversial since the growth of its source plant contributes to the destruction of rainforests. If you want to use this oil, choose to buy RSPO-certified palm oil.

Rice bran oil is rich in antioxidants and vitamin E. Like olive oil, it's so mild that you can make soap with 100% rice bran oil and it will still be suitable for sensitive skin.

Safflower oil is similar to canola oil. It's inexpensive, mild, and makes a softer bar of soap.

Shea butter makes soap feel silky and extra-moisturizing, just like cocoa butter. It contributes to the soap's hardness while providing a creamy lather.

Sunflower oil is rich in essential fatty acids and vitamin E and yet, it's quite inexpensive. It's possible to make soap with 100% sunflower oil but it will be soft and require more time to cure.

Sweet almond oil is a light oil that's suitable for all types of skin. It makes a soft bar of soap with a creamy lather.

Tallow, like lard, is from animal fat. It makes a hard bar of soap that's mild for the skin. It has little cleansing power, so it's usually paired with other oils.

Tamanu oil is a dark-colored oil with a nutty odor. It's moisturizing, rich in essential fatty acids, and easily absorbed into the skin.

Lye and Water

Lye is essential in soap making since soap is the product of the chemical reaction between oils and lye. Water dissolves and activates the lye and disperses it through the oils. When making soap, it's best to use distilled water.

Two types of lye are used in soap making: sodium hydroxide (NaOH) and potassium hydroxide (KOH). The latter is only used when making liquid soap.

If you want to make soap but are feeling uncomfortable about handling lye, you can still make soap following the melt-and-pour method.

Working with Lye

Lye is a strong chemical that can burn your skin if you come into contact with it. While it's dangerous, it shouldn't hold you back from making soap. By following these precautions, you'll be able to safely handle lye:

Before you start, remove all food from your work area and don't allow your kids or pets to get anywhere near it. Make sure that you always have quick access to running water and keep walkways clear.

Always wear your gloves and goggles when handling lye—even after mixing it with the oils. Avoid wearing short pants, short-sleeved shirts, or sandals.

Make sure that you're in a well-ventilated area when adding lye to water. Lye creates caustic steam, which you should avoid inhaling, as it dissolves in water. You can wear a face mask or wrap a bandana over your face for added protection.

Use distilled and chilled water. Always add lye to water. Never the other way around.

If your clothes get contaminated with lye, remove them immediately.

Always clean up spills and splashes right away.

Melt-and-Pour Soap Base

Soap bases are premade plain soaps that replace the oils, water, and lye in melt-and-pour recipes. They're usually named after the type of oil used to make it or a distinguishing ingredient.

Here are some of the most common soap bases:

White soap base – best for making soap with a simple look; adding color results to a pastel hue

Clear soap base – best for making vibrantly colored soap or soap with embeds or layers

Moisturizing soap base – made of a blend of oils that cleans and moisturizes the skin; includes shea butter soap base, goat's milk soap base, olive oil soap base, honey soap base, and hemp oil soap base

Soap Fragrance

Some soap makers prefer to keep their soap unscented, leaving it to smell like a clean, handmade soap or allowing the natural aroma of oils with unique fragrance to define the scent. After all, unscented soap is best for those with exceptionally sensitive skin. If you want to give your soap a particular scent, the most common way is to add cosmetic-grade fragrance oils or essential oils.

Essential Oil Vs Fragrance Oil

Essential oils are oils derived from different parts of a plant while fragrance oils are a mix of natural and synthetic chemical components formulated to mimic the smell of something natural or to have an entirely new smell.

Essential oils are 100% natural and aside from the scent, they often carry the health benefits of the plant they were extracted from. You can't expect a fragrance oil with the same scent as an essential oil to provide you with its aromatherapy benefits.

However, it requires hundreds of pounds of plant material to produce a pound of essential oil. This makes essential oils cost a lot. And if you're new to soap making, you may want to save that money for later, when you're already sure about what you're doing.

Fragrance oils offer a more affordable way to add scent to your soap. In fact, many of them are ridiculously cheap. They're also easier to find and you have more options to choose from.

Adding Fragrance

Before using any fragrance or essential oil, make sure that you read the description and instructions first. Even though essential oils are natural, they're still chemicals and you should always take caution when putting them in something that you will use on your body.

The amount of essential or fragrance oil you can add to your soap depends on the standard usage rate for that particular oil. Many experienced soap makers usually follow a *personal* maximum oil usage rate guideline based on the standards of regulatory bodies. Coming up with this guideline takes some research, calculation, and actual soap-making experience.

The recipes in this e-book follow a stricter guideline. You can add up to 0.48 ounces of essential oil for every pound of cold-process soap. For every pound of melt-and-pour soap, you can add up to 0.25 ounces of essential oil or 0.4 ounces of fragrance oil. If you want to use more oils for a stronger scent, make sure that you do your research first on that particular oil to ensure safety.

Colorants

Some of the oils used in making soap will impart a light yellow or creamy color. But if you want your soap to have a more vibrant color, you have several options to choose from. These range from store-bought pigments to plants that you might have in your garden.

Pigments are colorants in a powdered form available in two types—oxides and ultramarines. Even though they're synthetic, they're usually made with natural materials. Their colors also mimic those of naturally occurring things, like *iron oxide red*, commonly known as rust.

When coloring with pigments, premix the colorants with oil or liquid glycerin before adding to the soap batter. A teaspoon of pigment will give a pound of base oil a dark shade of color.

Mica colorants are powdered mica—a rock-forming mineral that can be peeled off in sheets—which are sterilized and combined with dyes or pigments to give them color. When used in clear soap, they give not just color but also a sparkly appearance.

Like pigments, it's best to premix mica with liquid to avoid clumps before adding to your soap. A teaspoon of mica colorant will give a pound of base oil a bold, dark shade.

F, D, and C dyes can be bought in powdered or liquid form. A liquid dye is added directly to the soap base. The dye in powdered form has to be mixed with a little water before adding to the soap.

Clays are usually used to make soap that detoxifies and lightly exfoliates the skin, but they also give the soap a natural color.

Herbs, flowers, and roots can be used to give your soap a natural color. Commonly used plant colorants are calendula petals (golden orange), madder root (pink), and alkanet root (purple).

Botanicals

Botanicals refer to flower, leaves, fruits, and roots that you can add to your soap to impart a natural color, make it more visually appealing, or provide exfoliation.

Dried fruits (lemon and orange slices) and spices (cinnamon sticks and apple spice) can give your soap scent- or holiday-themed designs.

Ground almonds, poppy seeds, and walnut shell powder are some of the additives you can use to create a scrubby soap.

Dried herbs and flowers can be used on top or in the interiors of your soap.

Ground turmeric, madder, and alkanet roots, when added directly to your soap, can give it a natural color.

Chapter 2: The Basics Of Soap Making

Like a base to making pancakes, you will require the liquid ingredients and the solid ingredients. Using chocolate or banana as a base will result in your pancakes becoming banana pancakes or chocolate pancakes. This is the same with soaps. The base that you select to use first, will determine the type of soap you are going to be making.

Soap Bases

Bases of soaps very greatly. The bases can be bought online or in stores in bulk. Bases are what your soap is going to be made of essentially.

There are those soaps whose base is glycerin. It is used as the first ingredient when you are making glycerin soap. A huge chunk is used before other ingredients are added to it.

The bases of glycerin soap can vary from vegetable to clear. In pour soaps, such a base is often used than in other soaps. Coming from animals and vegetables, glycerin has some sweetness to it, clear and quite thick.

The uses of glycerin are enormous for instance:

● It can be used in hydraulic equipment as a lubricant

● It is found in ink and cosmetics as well

● In the food we eat, as a substitute for sugar, it is used instead

● Used in jellies and canning food

When looking for a safe base, use glycerin. Though some people argue that glycerin soap uses alcohol and sugar. Some people think that glycerin soap has no lye in it, it is not true though. Handmade glycerin soap made from scratch can be extremely different from craft store glycerin soap.

Lard (which is rendered pork fat) is one of the popular bases used in the manufacturing industries. This is because it creates a creamy lather, the finished soap will be hard and it contains conditioning properties.

Many soaps now use fats and oils that have been mixed with lye (Sodium Hydroxide). Tallow (rendered beef fat), coconut oil and other solid oils are used in bar soaps to form the "bar" in soaps for it stay hard and to be able to withstand dissolving in water after being placed in a soap dish.

Soap chips are another kind of base that can be used. They are commonly used when making liquid soap. Making this type of base is pretty simple; cut up your soap into tiny pieces or buy one from the shop and grate it.

For recipes, the base has already been determined for you and you just have to go with the flow, but once you learn the art of making soap, you can make one using a base of your own choosing.

Ingredients

There are the key requirements that are needed in order for you to make your soap of choice. Essential oils are one requirement. Essential oils are extractions that are highly concentrated from various plants.

These oils are the most essential (see what I did there?) way of making your soap have a scent. To you as a potential soap maker, the number of essential oils at your disposal are too many and some soap makers mix several essential oils to get the scent they approve of.

Points to note:

● Not all essential oils out there are of benefit, thus be careful which oil you are going to add to your soap as an ingredient.

● Some oils are going to be irritable to your skin

● There are oils that will potentially create a problem when you use them for soap making, such as citrus oils.

Therefore, before you add any essential oil to your mix, do some research on which oils work best with what and how your skin will react to them when used.

There are fragrance oils as well, though most people can't for the life of them, tell or make the difference between them and essential oils.

Here is the difference between the two oils:

● Essential oils are extracted from plants while fragrance oils are made from either natural or synthetic ingredient to mimic the aroma of fruits.

• Essential oils can be extracted in large quantities while fragrance oils are only extracted in small quantities.

• Fragrance oils are not volatile oils while essential oils are volatile.

• Fragrance oils carry no therapeutic properties while essential oils, on the other hand, pack a ton of therapeutic properties.

• Essential oils are natural while fragrance oils are artificial, in translation, man-made.

The type of fruits that are found in essential oils are citrus fruits. The leaves of the plant and the rind of the fruit are the places where you can extract oil from. Lemon or orange rinds, we have all handled them, once we peel them the aroma we get is the essential oil; this aromatherapy is the purest you can get.

Now we will look at the different types of soaps:

a) Castile soap

As introduced in the first chapter, this is the oldest 'white soap" made in Italy. Though you don't need to be in Italy to make this soap, it is the easiest soap to make and a favorite among many.

The main ingredient is olive oil, making this soap really gentle and mild. A good soap to make for babies instead of buying soap from the store. Made from purely natural oils and no animal fat used, Castile soap is the most natural soap you can make for yourself and your baby(ies) if you don't have any, just be in the know.

You can use coconut oil or Jojoba oil to make Castile soap. It is safe for the planet, and with the current trend going green, the product is biodegradable. A win for us on our skin and a win for mother earth as we don't pollute it any further.

Other uses of Castile soap are:

● Use it to wash your hair. You will find out that you won't need to use a conditioner afterward.

● In liquid form, it can be used for pets as a shampoo.

● As a shaving lather, therefore, recommended for men as well.

● Women can use it as well for shaving their legs.

b)Milled soap

This is a form of industry process required equipment. The soap that is used here is diced into tiny pieces and left to dry. The next process is mashing the dried soap and rolling it to form a paste by applying pressure on the soap using metal rollers.

To achieve the desired shape, soap molds are used. The paste is placed into the soap molds. This type of soap is long lasting due to it being hard.

The make at home version of milled soap is what we are doing, without using the expensive and quite chic equipment. You first have to make soap, grate and wet it and finally and the scent you want. Then go all Hulk on the scented mix and mash them together.

Other people cook the grated soap and others add more water to it. An example of hand milling is soap balls.

c)Animal or vegetable soap

It all depends on whether you want to use tallow, that is from beef or lard from pigs, the decision is entirely up to you. With recommendations from others, it seems as if making soap from lard, makes the soap hard and of great quality as well.

Not everyone has high experience with an animal made soap, but it seems, if you are not squeamish, make yourself a batch of soap using these products.

d) Liquid soap

Similar to how Egyptians made their soap, using the ancient hot process. Instead of the standard Sodium Hydroxide, you use Potassium Hydroxide to create liquid soap.

When working using Potassium Hydroxide, you need to have patience, trucks and trucks of it. Trace is the one way to know if the batch you are making is all right, or ready for use; if you proceed too fast without waiting for the trace to appear, you can be misled into thinking the trace has already occurred only for it to disintegrate or separate again.

The method can take three to five hours, meaning your patience levels need to be super high, top of the notch. Act as if you are trying to trap something, for instance, a bird, you need to wait patiently for it to walk into the trap without you spooking it;

the bird is your consistency and the end result is you capturing the bird. Too fast, it fails too slow, you don't achieve your goal, which is soap.

Additives

In your kitchen, if you are there look through your cabinets, you'd be surprised to find the additives required to make soap.

Herbs can be bought from a store or you have grown some in your backyard and oatmeal is just a must have for most homes. Supplements, Aloe Vera, and vitamins can be found in health stores. If you have no clue where to get these; GOOGLE! It never disappoints, so I'm sure this time it will come through for you.

If you are the weird one and want your soap to have some scents that no one can pinpoint or as a prank to others (this can be a great way to get back at someone by swapping their soaps, you're welcome).

Go to ethnic stores, they will provide and cater to all your weird needs, in terms of soap.

Fats and Oils

They are both things we use on a daily basis, but at times getting the right fat or oil can be easy and hard at the same time. Some oils such as olive and vegetable oils are pretty easy to find, from your market store or the supermarket.

It is always difficult for you to find the right vegetable oils like coconut oil. To get it, you'd have to go to stores that specialize in vegetable oils. In health stores, it is guaranteed you will find almond oil and in the pharmacy close to you, castor oil will be in plenty. You can buy organic, to prevent you from having contaminated soap due to insecticides and pesticides used.

We are going to look into what you require to make the soap.

Chapter 3: Cold Process Soap-Simple Soap

The first thing you want to do is gather all of you ingredients, if you are just curious about making soap and are wanting to give it a try you can purchase the exact amounts of each ingredient needed but if you know you are going to make many batches of soap you should purchase the ingredients in larger quantities in order to save the most money possible.

This soap we are going to learn in this chapter is going to be a plain unscented soap. No frills just a nice bar of soap without a ton of chemicals. First you will need 18.5 ounces of olive oil. Using olive oil in your soap will give it a moisturizing effect on your skin. Next you need 12 ounces of coconut oil, this ensues the soap will lather well. 9 ounces of palm oil to ensure you have a nice firm bar of soap when you are finished. 1 ounce of Shea butter will help with moisturizing. 5.8 ounces of Lye. Now you may be saying Lye is a chemical, a corrosive, but the fact is that you cannot make soap without lye no matter what someone may tell you.

The trick is to use just the right amount of lye so that it completely dissolves into the oils you are using to make the soap with. That way you are not putting a bunch of chemicals on your skin. You want to have about 5 percent less lye in your soap than you do oils, this way you will end up with a smooth, mild bar of soap.

You will also need 13.5 ounces of water. If you are adding any type of essential oil to the soap you will need to get it as well.

With these ingredients you will get around 51 ounces of soap or 14 bars and you should end up paying about 50 cents per bar. That of course does not include if you add any essential oils for fragrance, this will of course make the price a bit higher but you should only be using a few drops of essential oils in the soap so even though essential oils are expensive they should not raise the price per bar too much.

Next we need to go over the different tools you will need to make your soap. The first thing you are going to need is a pair of safety glasses and rubber gloves. This is because you are going to be working with lye and it is very important to protect your eyes as well as your hands from any irritation the caused by the lye. You do not have to worry about this once the soap is made but while mixing it you want to make sure you are taking the necessary safety precautions.

You will also need a stick blender. This is going to cut your stirring time down from one hour to five minutes and will leave you with a smoother soap than hand stirring would.

A digital scale is needed to measure all of the ingredients precisely, and you will also need a cooking thermometer. The pot, bowls and spoons need to be stainless steel, make sure you are not using plastic or wooden spoon. You also need to ensure your pot you will be mixing in as well as the bowls are stainless steel because the lye will react to other pots including cast iron and you will not get the final product you desire.

You will need a large stainless steel pot, two stainless steel bowls and a stainless steel spoon. Next you will need some sort of soap mold. You can purchase different types of molds but I recommend starting out with a wooden rectangle. Many people just use a wooden plant box. You will not get anything fancy from this mold but you will be able to get nice bars of soap. Later if you decide you want to purchase different shape soap molds such as sea shells, you can do so.

You will need to make sure you have a card board box that will fit over whatever you are using for the soap mold, as well as freezer paper to line to mold with. The freezer paper will ensure the soap does not stick to the mold.

The last thing you will need is a large kitchen knife so that you will be able to cut your soap into bars once it is set. You will want to make yourself a soap making kit out of most of the supplies because you really don't want to cook a meal in something you have used lye in. I find that it works best if I keep my bowls, spoon and knife all in my large pot this way when I am ready to make soap everything is right there ready to do. I have also made it clear to the rest of the family that this is for soap making only and they are not to use it for cooking foods.

It may seem like this is going to cost you a lot of money if you do not already have these supplies on hand but if you don't mind using used items you can find most of this stuff at a resale shop. Since it is only going to be used for making soap you really don't have to worry about who owned it previously. The only thing I do recommend is that you take the time to deep clean each of the items when you get home because many of these items sit in resale shops for a long time and many people touch them before you buy them. You just want to make sure they are clean and germ free before you use them for your soap making.

You will probably have to purchase the lye online but most of these ingredients can be found locally. If you come across an ingredient in this book that you are having trouble finding just look on one of the many soap making supply stores online or even on Amazon. There is no reason for you to worry about not being able to find a specific ingredient and I am going to try through this entire book to make sure you are able to find all of the ingredients without too much work.

In the next chapter we are going to go over how to mix the ingredients as well as the final product.

Chapter 4: How To Make Glycerin Soap

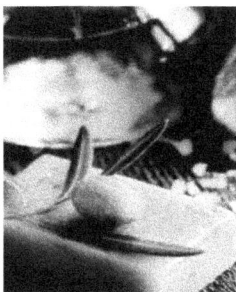

Step 1

Weigh the tallow, coconut, and castor oil according to your preferences. Melt the oil in a slow cooker or oven, weigh the distilled water and lye. Pour the lye into the water and stir until it's dissolved.

Step 2

Add the lye mixture to the oil, use your mixer to mix properly until it thickens a little, mix until you reach trace. Cook for 3 hours, weigh the alcohol, weigh the glycerin, then add the alcohol and glycerin to the cooked mixture and stir.

Step 3

Mix with your mixer, then cover and cook for 30mins longer, weigh the sugar and water, then mix them together to make sugar syrup. Add the sugar syrup to the soap. Test for translucence, fill the mixture into your molds and allow it to cool.

The Making of Pomegranate Soap

Step 1

Pour oil mixture into a container, add in 'room temperature' lye water, add in your palm oil, then mix with a whisk until mixture reaches a thin trace, once done add in grapefruit and lemongrass fragrance oil.

Step 2

Add synstar red mica, mix with a whisk and add in your pomegranate, add mica again, then add in pomegranate into each cavity of a sanitized mold.

Step 3

Tap to remove any bubble, sprinkle on more pomegranate if you wish, then leave the soap to harden for about 24-48 hours. Once ready, pull the mold away from the soap. And gently remove soap from mold; the soap needs to cure for about 4 weeks.

Soap from Orange Zest

You need a soap base, orange juice, orange peel, aloe vera gel, rose water.

Step 1

Dry the orange peel, make sure the orange peel is cut into small pieces, blend it till it is in smooth powder, then separate big particles from powder using a sieve.

Step 2

Cut your soap base in small pieces, boil the water, melt the soap base using double boiling method, add two spoons of orange juice, and stir very well, then add one spoon of aloe vera gel and stir.

Step 3

Add orange peel the small particles of it and stir, then add two drops of rose water. Put the big particles of the orange peel into an empty mold and pour your soap mixture into it. Allow it to dry.

Mango Butter Soap

Step 1

Get your mango; after blending in the mango seed, you go ahead to add 500 grams of shea butter and 200grams of your mango butter already blended. Please try to avoid mold; you have to dry the mango parts and let it dry. After blending to be powder, let it dry a little because the inner part has some liquid.

Step 2

Next, you are going to blend the whole thing together to become creamy. I mean, fluffy, cream that they can spread on top of bread, or you can spread on your skin because it is going to make your skin to become moisturizing.

Step 3

After blending through, put it in a jar or any container or your mold. So Allow it to sit; it will solidify, so you can put it in the refrigerator for it to form.

Chapter 5: Soap Makers Come And Go

Another way that openings continually present themselves for new soap marketers just results from natural attrition.

People stop selling soap for all kinds of reasons.

Some people just get tired of the work for example. Don't forget that a soap business, as opposed to a soap hobby, means that the more success you have, the more soap must be made. It turns to work at some point.

Face To Face Works For Soap Marketing

Many ways can be used to move soap. One way that continues to work is to get in front of people and show them what you have.

Basically, building relationships with people by talking with them works wonders to get people to try what you have to offer. Especially if you can talk to many potential customers in a short time, you have a great chance to gain new customers.

It's The Follow-up For More Sales

Then here's the key. It's the follow-up part that many soap sellers fail at miserably, or rather they don't even try. Finding a new customer is the hardest and most expensive part of marketing. Once you have a customer, it's necessary to follow up with that customer and offer them more of what they already want. That's easy enough with a little home-produced brochure or catalog, and maybe even a website too.

It's true that starting a soap business is easier than starting many other home-based businesses. The competition is stiff, but it may still work for you. There are several reasons why making soap can still produce profits, in spite of the large number of competitors.

Discover How Fun Soap Making is For You

Looking for a new hobby to keep you busy? There are several options that you can try but soap making is a very interesting one. Imagine using soaps that you, yourself has customized. Wouldn't that be a great idea? Rather than using the old, boring white soap bars that you use, you can now have different soaps everyday.

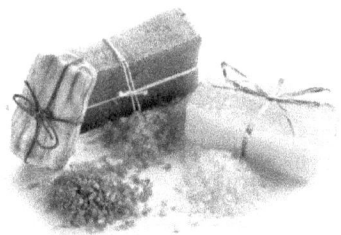

People are very much into this because it allows them to be very creative. There are different ways to actually make soaps. It all depends on how you want to make your soaps. There is the melt and pour method, hot process, cold process and handmilled process of making soaps.

If you plan to start with this activity now, the first things that you have to know are the substances that are used to make these soaps. Soaps are primarily made from mixing fats and oils. This is called the saponification process. You can use fats from animal or even vegetable. Other ingredients also include color, essentials oils and dyes. Just mix everything to get the ideal soap that you want to make.

If are trying out soap making for the first time, you can start with the melt and pour method. This is a simple process to make since everything is ready for you. You just have to melt the soap base to make liquid soap. The next step is adding the additives to alter your soap. Pour the soap into the molds and let it harden. This is how easy this is.

Probably the cold process of soap making is a hassle-free method that you can try. First, it is important to mix the lye into water. Once this is done, add the fat in this mixture until it forms an emulsion. The additives go in next so add whatever you want to in the mixture. Cure this in the mild for 3 days until t is hard enough to cut. Once the soaps are solid, you have to cure the soap for an additional 3 weeks before you can practically use it.

The hot process is a modified method for handmade soaps. Compared to the cold process, this requires heating of the ingredients. Both the lye-water and the oils must be heated prior and after adding them. Continuous stirring will mix the ingredients all together. The additives must be added in the soap before transferring into molds. The advantage of this is that the soaps that have hardened can immediately be used.

Rebatching soaps is an interesting method of making soaps. You have to grate old soaps that you want to recycle. Add in water to dissolve the soap previously made. Melt the soap and water mixture until it becomes liquid. Colorants and other additives go in the melted mixture. Once these have hardened in the molds, that's the time that you can actually use the soaps.

We all use soaps whenever we take a bath. It will really be very exciting if we can actually use a new type of soap each time. With soap making as a hobby, you are allowed to be very creative.

Soap Making - Finding Perfect Fragrances:

Working with scents, whether natural or synthetic, can be one of the most rewarding and one of the most frustrating aspects of soap making. When deciding how to scent your soaps, there are many factors that that you must weigh. In this article, we'll look at the advantages and disadvantages of using fragrance oils vs. essential oils in soap and we'll talk about how to test your scents to find which ones work best for you. There are many advantages of using fragrance oils in soap making. Some of these are:

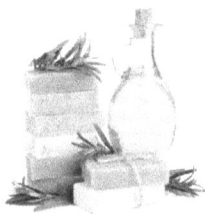

Low cost: Fragrance oils, in most cases, cost much less that their natural essential oil counterparts. Because of this, using fragrance oils makes sense in many cases.

Safe to use on skin: Some natural essential oils can actually harm the skin. Cosmetic grade fragrance oils are designed to be used in skin care products.

Can obtain scents otherwise impossible to obtain with essential oils: Many scents do not exist in nature. If you want your soap to smell like pear, mango, or tomato, using fragrance oils is the only way to go.

Can add colors to your soaps: Some fragrance oils, in particular vanilla, will add color to your soap, if added during the soap making process. Depending on what you expect, this may or may not be an advantage.

Disadvantages of using fragrance oils:

Some react negatively to cold-processed soaps: One of the most frustrating things that can happen to a soap maker is to discover a beautiful fragrance oil and to add it to a soap batch during the soap making process only to have it curdle the soap. Unfortunately, some fragrance oils are just not compatible with cold-processed soaps. The only way to obtain these scents is to add them to soap, after the soap making process.

Formulas can vary from one manufacturer to another: You may like a scent from one company, and find the same scent from another company at a lower price. Don't expect these two fragrance oils to respond the same way in your soap making process. Test, test, test before ordering large amounts of any fragrance oil, because their formulas will differ from one company to another.

Can add colors to your soaps: Depending on your perspective, this may or may not be a disadvantage. I have read many accounts of soap makers who complain that vanilla fragrance oil turns soap brown. However some large scale bath companies sell dark brown vanilla soap. I guess it depends on your perspective.

For those who prefer using essential oils there are also several advantages and disadvantages to weigh: Advantages of using essential oils:

Natural: Many people are concerned with the invasion of synthetic ingredients into foods and cosmetics. For those who want natural cosmetics, essential oils are the way to go.

Therapeutic Value: In addition to scent, many essential oils have natural properties which can treat skin and hair problems.

Disadvantages of using essential oils

Many are too expensive to use in soap: My biggest gripe about essential oils is that many are too expensive to use in soap (or in other cosmetics for that matter).

Some have a limited shelf life and must be used quickly after purchase: Most essential oils are processed using steam-distillation. This procedure uses heat and helps preserve the essential oils, But cold-pressed citrus oils retain components that can cause these oils to turn rancid quickly.

The price fluctuates from one season to another. Since essential oils are derived from plants, the price is affected by weather, by crop yield, and by other things out of the control of the soap maker.

The choice is up to each individual soap maker about what to use for scent. Your choice will be a reflection of your needs and the needs of those who use your soap.

After you decide which fragrance or essential oil you are interested in adding to your collection, you need to do some testing to make sure it will work in your products. always order a small amount first and test it for the following four items:

Does the fragrance oil or essential oil smell nice? Some smell nice, others don't. If you don't like the smell of your test amount, don't order any more.

Does the fragrance oil or essential oil discolor your products? Sometimes certain fragrance oils, such as vanilla, will slightly or drastically discolor your products. Always test a small amount of your fragrance oil in your lotions and soaps before ordering a larger amount.

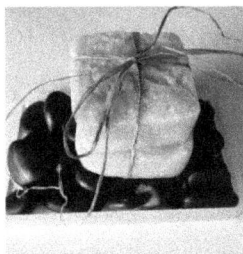

Does the fragrance oil or essential oil work in soap? If you make handmade soaps, always test a small amount of a new scent in a small batch of soap. Check to see whether or not the scent causes your test batch of soap to curdle or react strangely.

Does the scent in your test batch fade with time? Some scents work beautifully in products, but a few weeks later will fade to nothing, even when your product is enclosed in plastic. This can be very frustrating. If this happens, try another manufacturer or vendor to see if you can get a similar fragrance oil with a scent that lasts longer.

Testing will help you to choose the perfect fragrances for your soap.

Keeping it Healthy

It is believed that soap probably had its origins in sap from different plants. These were referred to as soap plants and one could take the roots of the plant, crush them in water and the result would be a rich lather. These plants still exist today but are no longer used in their raw form.

Plants that fell into the category of soap plants were soap bark, soap wort and a plant that was called soap berry. All of these plants would produce a foam that could also be used as a lather. In ancient times these plants were also used to catch fish as the lather could immobilize them, thereby making them easier to catch.

Much later people found that certain fats could react when combined with the alkalies found in the ashes of burned wood. It would cause the fat to saponify different compounds such as sodium sterate as well as potassium sterate.

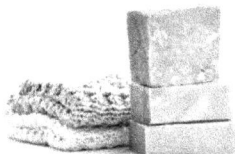

In today's world soap is now made from a combination of fats and oils that interact with lye. Oils such as coconut, palm, tallow or rendered beef and lard which is rendered fat from pork are commonly used in bar soap and are normally hard soaps that do not dissolve easily in water.

Castile soaps are mainly made using olive oil, normally the purest you can find, and yields a soap that is known for being very mild and soft on your skin. This is a favorite soap for many because of its healing properties for your skin.

There is also a process in soap making that is called super fatting. Once the interaction with lye is complete the soap tends to have some fat remaining. This soap is normally easier to cut and feels very smooth on your skin. The lye is completely burned off and none remains that could cause any kind of irritation to the skin of the user. This type of soap is also very low in alkaline.

Glycerin is also another popular ingredient in soap making and many will use it to make transparent soaps. Glycerin is also one of the main ingredients that you rarely find in commercial soaps as it is usually removed. This is one reason that commercially bought soaps are so hard on your skin and often contribute to skin dryness.

Soaps that are sold commercially usually contain ingredients such as sodium tallowate, sodium palmate and a number of other ingredients that are not naturally produced. This is one of the main reasons that people prefer to buy homemade soaps as they realize the health value of using these soaps as well as the value to their skin.

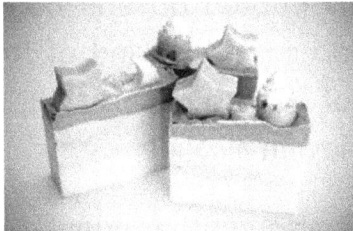

People also like to buy natural soaps as not only do they like to use them to bath with but in many cases the soaps are great as a shampoo. Naturally made soaps will not contain harmful ingredients and harsh chemicals.

One of the fun soap ingredients is using essential oils. People love to use them separately for a pure scent as well as combining them to make a combination of scents. Soap makers love to experiment with essentials oils and it helps to lend a certain amount of creativity to the soap making process.

Another soap making ingredient that people love to work with is different colors that are produced from many different sources. From Crayola crayons to pigments from different plants the choices are endless.

But in the end, the great thing about soap is that these use basic ingredients, naturally produced and much healthier for the person using them or purchasing them.

The art of liquid soap making is probably one of the easiest ways to make your own soap at home. It's easy because melting down old pieces of soap, or even an entire bar is quick and simple. Liquid soap in it's simplest form is bar soap that has had water added to it, until you have nothing but liquid left. The only tools you will require are a pot, a measuring cup and a stove to heat everything.

You can also take it up a notch yet still keep it simple, by adding some fragrances to your soap or essential oils along with a bit of coloring. For the most part though, liquid soaps are usually put into a container where you use a hand pump and for the most part these are not normally see-through, so color does not necessarily have to be a consideration.

The first thing you do for liquid soap making is to take a bar of soap, or even old pieces, and grate them as finely as possible. When they get too small use a knife to cut them up, making sure to get it as fine as possible. The next step is to put the grated soap into a cup with measurements on the side and add water to equal the amount of grated soap.

The most difficult part of liquid soap making is the diluting process. If you use too little liquid then you may see your soap start to form a skin or it globs up in the bottle. If you add too much liquid then you won't see a good lather.

It's important to make sure you follow your recipe to the letter or you will run into problems. For the most part liquid soap making is the easiest of all the soaps that you can make at home. Knowing this, you will probably be fine and your recipe will work each time.

One of the most common reasons these days to use liquid soap is to help stop the spread of germs. With the recent flu scare, people in Mexico City started using anti-bacterial soap and washing their hand as often as possible. The result, besides helping to stop the spread of the flu germ, was a forty percent decrease in gastrointestinal problems. Nowadays it should be common practice for every sink to have some kind of liquid soap on the side for cleanliness as well as protection during flu seasons.

With liquid soap you can add any number of essential oils that also serve as anti-bacterial agents. Oregano and tea tree oil are both great for this, but there are also many others to choose from. You can even blend them with other essential oils for an even more pleasant smell and yet still have an effective product. One note of caution.

It is not advisable to use perfumed fragrances in combination with essential oils and still expect to have an effective product. You also need to take into consideration that if guests are using the liquid soap, and they have skin problems, then perfumed soap may not be to their liking. For guest bathrooms it is suggested that you stick to all-natural ingredients whenever possible.

One thing that recently has become very popular is liquid face soap. My favorite is goat's milk. A simple recipe is to reduce your water content by about eight ounces, then add 0.2 ounces of potassium hydroxide for every twelve ounces of goat's milk. This will cause the goat's milk fat to saponify. It's that simple and you will have a fantastic face soap that can easily be used on a daily basis.

The main thing to remember with liquid soap making is that it is the simplest technique around and probably the most foolproof. It's a great way to get started making soap, or introducing your children to the wonderful world of soapmaking at home.

Hot Process Soap Making - Your Guide For Homemade Soap

Hot process soap making is simply a variation of the cold process method of soap making. Making soap via the hot process method is at times the method preferred by soap makers because they have the option of creating soaps from scratch. In addition, this method is combined with the science of creating the soap from beginning to end. Furthermore, cooking the soap thoroughly eliminates the long cure time for soap as compared to the cold process soap making method.

When using the hot process method, the soap ingredients are added to a cooking vessel and placed over some type of heat source. The most commonly used vessels are a stove, microwave, or even a crock pot. After being "cooked", the mixture is poured into a mold and the excess water is allowed to evaporate. Once the mixture is entirely cooled it be may be un-molded and used.

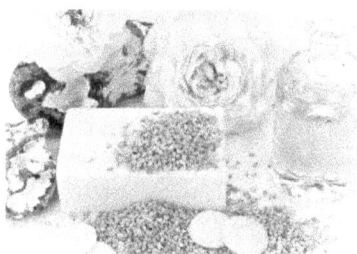

The hot process soap method is an excellent choice for individuals who want to customize soap recipes to include a wide range of the base ingredients of their choice but do not want to wait for the extended cure time for the soap to be completed.

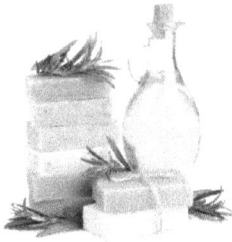

While the hot process soap making is simple, it is a technique that requires practice and patience. Many expert soap makers agree that it is best attempted after an individual has mastered the cold process soap making technique as well as the melt and pour methods of soap making.

The following instructions will provide you with the necessary techniques to employ with the hot process method recipe. Note: Olive oil should not be used with the hot process soap method because of the delicate composition of olive oil soaps.

Before starting the hot process method, make sure you have all of the necessary equipment ready to use and the ingredients prepared that are called for in the recipe.

You will need the following equipment for the hot process method:

One large pot

A heat source. Use a stove, double boiler, crock pot or microwave safe container and a microwave.

A soap mold and freezer paper or waxed paper. The freezer paper or waxed paper is used for lining the mold. If you do not line the mold it will be very difficult to remove the soap. Wooden soap molds work best for hot process soap.

Add your water to the pot and then heat it gently. Slowly add lye to the water and dissolve. Important note: never add water to lye. Always add the lye to the water.

Add the fats in the recipes such as: coconut oil, sesame oil, and shea butter.

when the soap begins to form inside the cooking utensil.

After saponification is complete, take the soap off of the heat source and then use a spatula to assist in pouring the mixture into soap molds that have been lined with freezer or wax paper. When using freezer paper, make sure you have it shiny side facing up.

Allow your soap to set up and when it is time to remove it from the mold, gently un-mold the soap from the molds. The soap will be slightly sticky, but rest assured that this is normal. However, after it cures for about three to four weeks it will dry out enough to remove the stickiness from its texture.

The hot process method of soap making is a combination of art and science. Find some recipes and try your hand today!

Chapter 6: Four Methods Of Soap Making

There are actually just four basic approach of making soap at home. Those are:

☐ Melt and Pour

☐ Cold Process

☐ Hot Process

☐ And Rebatching

Now, let's start discussing the two most common and popular methods of making soap:

☐ Melt and Pour

☐ Cold Process

Melt And Pour Process

Melt and Pour Soap Making is perhaps the easiest and safest method of making soap because you will not really get in contact with lye especially if you are allergic on it.

This method is just basically like making a cake with the use of a cake mix.

In this method, you purchase a pre-made blocks of unscented and uncolored soap bases from a particular soap supplier. You'll then melt the soap base in microwave, or just heat it on a stove. After completely melting the soap, add the desired color, fragrance, or additives. Pour the mixture in a mold, and surprisingly, you're done! You can now use the soap whenever you want as long as it completely hardens.

Here's a basic process:

☐Find a clean workspace. Of course make sure you already got a microwave or anything that can serve as melter.

☐A heat-resistant container for melting the pre made soap base

☐ Spoons or whisks for mixing and stirring

☐ Measuring spoons

☐ Get your desired color, fragrance, or additives

☐ And a mold

☐ Pour the mixture into the mold

☐ Wait for the mixture to harden

And you're finished. Simple, right?

But let's see some pros and cons of this method.

PROS:

☐ Frugal way of starting to make soap

☐ Far from possible harm of lye mixture

☐ No need for various ingredients

☐ Fast results

CONS:

☐ You don't have control over your ingredients because they are pre-made

☐ Pre-made ingredients are not really natural

☐Basically, your finished product will be only as good as the pre-made you bought

Cold Process

Now, let's go with the cold process of making soap.

If the previous method uses pre-made ingredients to make soap, the cold process begins from scratch. You manipulate every ingredients you have that goes into the mixing container, and you have the choice to make a finished product as natural as possible. Obviously, the setup would be a little complex, and you also need to learn some techniques to craft your soap perfectly.

Now let's start. To start the cold process, you begin by heating your chosen essential oils up until 100 degrees. Then gradually add the lye water mixture. After mixing them for a couple of minutes, you can now add some additional stuff, like color, fragrance, and additives, and you pour the mixtures into a mold.

It will take for about one whole day to harden the raw soap, and around 4 weeks to cure before use. Ultimately, it is called a cool process, because you let it cool and get cured until ready to use.

Now, what are the pros and cons of Cold process?

PROS:

☐ You have full control over the ingredients

☐ You have unlimited variations

☐You can make your soap as natural as possible

CONS:

☐You must know how to handle lye

☐More ingredients, means more cost

☐You need to wait longer before you can use your soap

In the field of making soap, you must always remember that there are various kinds of processes and methods used.

To sum it up, there's the melt and pour approach on which you uses a pre-made base to make your own soap and there's the cold process on which you have full access over your ingredients. It's up to you what you choose though.

Of course, there's some complex methods of making soap such as the saponification process on which you use the own heat of your soap and saponifies it overnight.

There's also this so called hot process, on which you mixes all the essential oils and lye and then you add extra heat to jump start the saponification phase, and ultimately cooks your soap to finished the process.

And lastly, you mustn't forget that there's a method called, rebatching on where you take soap that has already been processed and giving it a new character by grating it, and melting it, then you add additional fragrances, colors, or additives that you desire. It's basically similar to melt and pour method. The only difference is that rebatching doesn't use a general pre-made soap base but a typical soap over the counter.

But regardless of countless methods out there, sometimes it is just always better to stick with the traditional and basic approach of making soap especially if you are just starting out (i.e. melt and pour, and the cold process).

Chapter 7: Equipment

Looking for soap making supplies? You've been thinking about it for awhile. Wondering if you should spend the extra money and if it will be worth it. And I can honestly tell you that yeah, it's definitely worth it!

Sure you could spend a fortune buying all the latest and greatest soapmaking gadgets but seriously, you can fully equip your soapmaking kitchen very easily without breaking your wallet.

Before you spending a single peny, take a look around your kitchen. You might be surprised to find you that a lot of the tools and equipment are probably already in your kitchen. If not, check your nearby thrift store, dollar store or discount retailer. The more bargains you find, the more money you will have left over for the soap making ingredients.

Just keep in mind that whatever you confiscate from your kitchen cannot be used for anything but soap making again.

The Basic Soap Making Supplies List

Tools Needed for Making Cold-Process Soap

An immersion blender, it does an hour worth of stirring in about 5 minutes, which ensures a better result. It sturdy, and with the push of a button the stick detaches from the handle for washing it.

Precise measuring of ingredients by weight is essential, especially for smaller batches.

Stainless steel is recommended for your soapmaking pot. The lye will react to an aluminum, teflon-coated, or cast iron pot.

A couple of bowls for measuring and mixing. At least one needs to be stainless steel or pyrex, so it can withstand high heat. Use stainless steel, glass, or plastic for your bowls and spoons. Do not use any made of aluminum or wood.

For measuring and stirring. Use stainless spoons. Do not use wooden spoons.

A cooking thermometer.

wood or plastic box. Your soap mold can be any container. You can even use milk cartons or pringle cans. It is up to your imagination

o line the soap mold, so the soap will not stick.

(large enough to cover the soap mold.)

Use a regular kitchen knife with a large blade.

Safety equipment

Rubber gloves, apron or old clothes and safety goggles. Rubber gloves will protect your hands from becoming irritated by the lye.As you make more batches of soap, you'll tailor your tools to fit your particular soap making style, but this is a good basic setup that should accommodate most soap projects.

Chapter 8: The Process

Do not be too prescriptive in your soap-making. Follow basic soap recipes but, just as you would in baking, change certain ingredients to suit yourself. After you have made a few batches and you are feeling confident, you can even use some of the ingredients in your kitchen and substitute them for some of the ingredients on the list. Having balanced ingredients will ensure the best result. Remember, even too much of a good thing may produce a poor result.

Melt and Pour:

If you are a little daunted by the cold process, you could consider the melt and pour option first because then the soap has a pre-made base. It is basically a plain block made traditionally from glycerin or white coconut oil (as they are the easiest to melt) to which you can add fragrance and any of your own touches to personalize your soap. So, if gift making is your intention, you can craft a soap without coming into contact with chemicals. The process is also quick and satisfying.

Soaps made using the melt and pour process do not last as long as once in use but they are still much appreciated.

You will need:

A plain block of soap or possibly a few which you can melt together.

Essential oils, fragrances and colors

Method:

You will need a large double-boiler (although you can melt the soap in the microwave but will have less control over it) and your essential oils and any colors or fragrances. Then you will just need your imagination to create a unique, most personal bar of soap.

Extreme care should be taken around children as the soap mixture will reach a very high temperature.

Break the soap bar into chunks and place over boiling water in the double boiler. Melt the soap.

Allow to cool and add the fragrances, essential oils (6g to 8 g per 150g soap) and any coloring. A few drops of color will make for a pretty, pastel bar of soap.

CARE: Do not use food coloring as it may stain the skin.

Stir the mixture taking care not to allow bubbles to form – do not stir too vigorously. Rubbing alcohol can be used to eliminate bubbles if they do form on your soap. Spray the rubbing alcohol onto your mixture.

Pour the soap mixture into your prepared mold and spray again with the rubbing alcohol to ensure a smooth finish.

For the best results allow your soap to form at room temperature. You may place it in the fridge but this will reduce the fragrance.

Once it has hardened, remove it from the mold and use plastic wrap to prevent evaporation or to protect from humidity.

Handy tips:

Do not use fragrances or color if you have sensitive skin as they will irritate it.

Use a petroleum jelly inside the mold for ease of removal

If you use pieces of silver / aluminum foil as your mold, you can shape the soap into various shapes using your hands. Wear rubber gloves and ensure that the soap has cooled to a manageable level.

The Cold Process:

When you are ready to do everything yourself, then you can follow the traditional "cold process" for making soap. The only heat used in the process is that required for the oils.

The vocabulary that you need to familiarize yourself with, especially for the cold process, contains words like

Trace – Trace can be seen when your soap resembles a thick custard. On removing the stick blender, the trail left behind is trace. The different consistencies of trace may be light, medium and heavy, depending on the desired result.

The gel phase – not all soaps go through this. If you cool the soap quickly, it will eliminate this phase and the result will be soap with a matt rather than a shiny finish.

Curing ensures a hard, long-lasting soap. Cure for an average of four to six weeks to ensure that, once it is used in the shower, for example, it lasts a sufficient length of time.

Saponification- This is the chemical reaction that takes place. Once the soap has been poured into the mold, this takes about 24 to 48 hours.

Your soap needs to have certain basic functions and meet certain basic requirements to ensure you are not disappointed with the end result:

For stability, and to make your soap hard, use lard or sustainable palm oil.

For those all essential bubbles or a lather, use coconut oil or castor oil

To ensure your soap does not dry your skin, add sunflower oil, olive oil, canola or rapeseed oil.

For a more luxurious feel and good moisturizing qualities add cocoa butter, shea butter or almond oil.

As quantities differ, using percentages is a useful way of apportioning quantities. So for the perfect beginner (cold process) bar of soap, work along the following lines:

25% sustainable palm oil

25% coconut oil

25% olive oil

10% canola (rapeseed) oil

10% sunflower oil

5% castor oil

When you have perfected your soap-making, you will be able to use the percentages to alter the recipe; say, if you want to make a larger quantity.

The ingredients are ideally weighed but, due to conversion difficulties, for beginners, it is recommended to work with cups, as follows. A standard cup is 250 ml:

¾ cup sustainable palm oil

1¼ cups coconut oil

¼ cup cocoa butter

1¼ cup olive oil

¼ cup castor oil

¾ cup lye

3/8 cup (that is just less than half a cup) sunflower oil

300 ml water

2 tblsp lightly ground lavender buds

3 tsp orange essential oil

5 tsp lavender essential oil

It will take about 20 to 30 minutes to prepare and 30 minutes to cook. The result will be about one and a half kg of soap.

Chapter 9: Expert Soap Making Techniques

Are you feeling kind of level and exhausted requiring something to involve your interests? Tired of playing web recreations for quite a long time and no enthusiasm for anything on TV? Leisure activities can be the solution for your quandary; it positively was the response for me. My primary issue is that I need to do it all, I need to attempt each specialty and diversion I keep running over!

There are side interests that can fill a double need by giving you real wage from your leisure activity. Making cleansers and shower salts is a pastime that can be sheltered, modest and enthralling... also it can pay for itself on the off chance that you offer your completed items.

In this article, I am going to furnish you with regulated direction alongside formulas for things that you can make and use to improve your home, give as blessings or even offer a benefit.

To discover what cleanser making includes, begin just by starting with a simple formula, Chocolate soap is a decent starter and here is the thing that you require:

12 oz ground cleanser

5 oz water

1/4 glass moment cocoa powder

1/8 oz Chocolate Scent oil

Join your ground cleanser and water in a pot and set on medium warmth; When the soap has dissolved the consolidated cocoa powder and chocolate aroma; Blend well and after that pack into molds and permit to sit until totally solidified.

When you are prepared stride it up we will start with making glycerine cleansers... this is the thing that you should make Apple Tart Cleanser:

4oz. Clear, Unscented Glycerine Cleanser

1 Tablespoon Fluid Cleanser

One teaspoon Fluid Glycerine

1/2 teaspoon Apple Aroma Oil

2 Drops Red Nourishment Shading

1/2 teaspoon Ground Cinnamon

In the first place you dissolve cleanser in little dish over moderate warmth or in a glass container in the microwave; Include Fluid Cleanser and glycerine and blend delicately however well; Include scent and/or shading; Include cinnamon and mix; Permit to remain for two or three minutes, sufficiently only to begin to thicken so when you mix again the cinnamon will be all the more uniformly appropriated; Fill molds. Permit to set totally (in or out of cooler). At the point when totally set you can wrap your cleanser in plastic wrap, treat cellophane sacks additionally work extremely well.

Another sort of glycerin cleanser that is intriguing to make is Apricot Freesia, and this is the thing that you will require:

1 lb White Glycerin Cleanser Base

12 Drops Enormous Shading Canary Yellow

11 Drops Enormous Shading Red

One t. Apricot Freesia FO

Elements For "Whipped Cream" Topping:

4 oz White Glycerin Cleanser Base

¼ t. Apricot Freesia FO

To begin with you soften cleanser base for tart in a twofold heater; After it is totally liquefied, include shading and aroma;

Empty blend into a biscuit tin and permit to solidify; Expel from tin; Melt cleanser base for garnish and include a shake of Shimmer Dust; Utilizing an electric blender, blend until thickened and bubbly; Shower with rubbing liquor and spoon the fixing onto the tarts and permit a portion of the fixing to keep running over sides; Top with a dash of Shimmer Dust (discretionary)

Being one who does a great deal of stimulating and investing energy with kids, Treat Cutter Cleanser was an absolute necessity! The making of this cleanser obliges one to be innovatively free and is a decent specialty for youngsters, with grown-up supervision obviously.

Dissolve and Pour cleanser base(opaque)

Fragrance (discretionary)

Shading (must be fluid, similar to gels)

treat sheet (must have no less than a 1/2 in. edge on it)

blade (to twirl your hues!)

treat cutters

In the first place you will need to dissolve down the cleanser base and aromas; You can give the principle support a shading in the event that you wish or abandon it white; Pour the base on the treated sheet and include hues and twirl every one of them over - this is the place you get the opportunity to be inventive! When this dries, pop the square of cleanser out of the treated sheet. Use handle cutters to cut up the soap.

There are heaps of various things you can do with this for the case you can make...

Christmas Cleanser: Twirl red and green into white and utilize treat cutters;

Confection Stick Cleanser: Twirl red into white with peppermint fragrance and sweet stick cutters;

Easter/Spring: Twirl various pastels and discover some fun treat cutters;

fourth of July: Enthusiastic white cleanser with a beautiful red and blue whirl (locate a pleasant star cutter!)

So you see your choices are boundless to the extent what you can make and offer on the off chance that you crave!

Chapter 10: Cold Process Soap Making

Cold process soap making will take you a little time, from half an hour to one and a half hours depending on the complexity of the recipe. At cold process, from scratch, soap becomes smooth, flat and beautiful. The scope of creativity here is not limited: you can make soap with swirls - whimsical swirls, striped soap, with different accents, etc. To decorate the soap there are variety of techniques that are used for working with such fluid and plastic materials. You have certainly noticed the similarity with decorative manicure.

On the other hand, this method has a disadvantage: before using the soap must ripen at least three weeks.

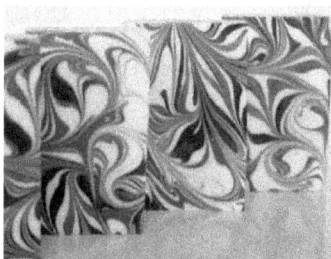

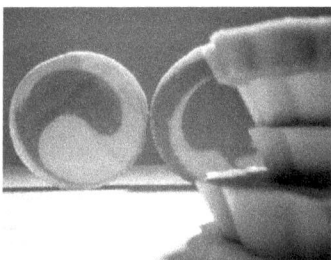

Do not forget that the safety rules should be kept when working with alkali - above all! So, all the tools are ready, oils and additives are selected, the recipe for soap making is ready too ...

Step 1. Cover the work surface and the floor around the work area with oilcloth or newspapers of several layers. Prepare all the tools and utensils. If the mold you are going to use is a wooden box, grease it with repellent paper or parchment.

Step 2. Weigh oils for basic recipe: put solid oils and waxes (if there are in the recipe) in a bowl for the water bath, and liquid vegetable oils leave for a while in a separate container. Prepare and measure all that you will use in the soap further: useful additives, dyes, essential oils, fragrances, etc.

Step 3. Weigh liquid (or ice) for alkaline solution in a glass or a heat resistant plastic container. For the preparation of the alkaline solution it is very convenient to use heat-resistant glass beaker and a wand. Place a glass with liquid in the sink, fill it with a little cold water, you can also put ice cubes in it - this will avoid excessive heating of the solution. In a separate container weigh alkali - plastic container out of sour cream, yogurt, or a disposable cup will perfectly do.

Step 4. Put solid oils for melting over the heat. For convenience, place there the thermometer - this will allow you to control the temperature and prevent oil overheating. While oil melts, make the alkaline solution. Add alkali in small portions into a glass with liquid, stirring constantly.

Important: add alkali to the liquid, and not vice versa!

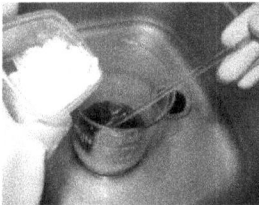

Water or decoction of herbs will immediately get turbid.

Water solution

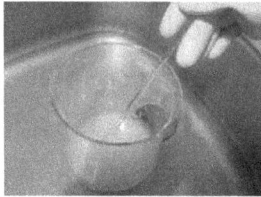

Solution on decoction of herbs

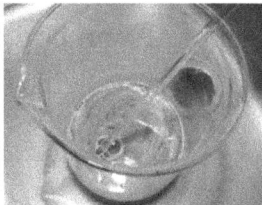

While dissolution of alkali reacts with water releasing a lot of heat, so be careful: the glass becomes too hot. A release of harmful fumes is also possible, so do not lean over the glass.

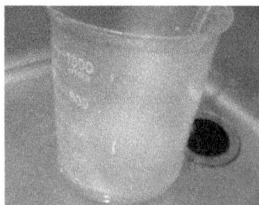

After complete dissolution of the alkali, aqueous solution again becomes clear. Periodically measure the temperature of the solution with a second thermometer.

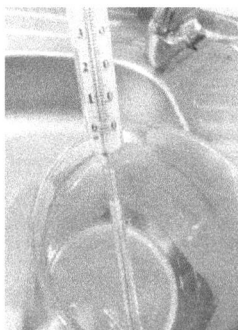

Step 5. Now it is necessary that the temperature of oil and the alkaline solution would be approximately equal with the difference of 2-3 degrees. The optimal temperature range for mixing: 30-70 degrees Celsius.

When solid oils melt, add the earlier delayed liquid oils – it will additionally cool oil mixture. To cool oil mixture you can also put it in a saucepan with cold water container. If together with hard wax oils you drown solid oils, then let the mixture cools down naturally, otherwise the wax at sharp cooling will stick to the walls of the ware and you will have to re-warm the mixture.

To cool the alkaline solution, add ice-cubes into the sink.

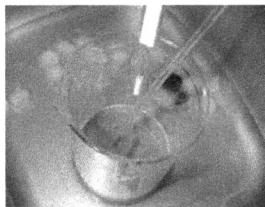

Step 6. When the desired temperature is reached, pour the alkaline solution in the oil very carefully, stirring gently with a spoon or blender. Oil mixture will immediately become turbid. Now start whisking the mixture with blender: gently without lifting it to avoid splashing.

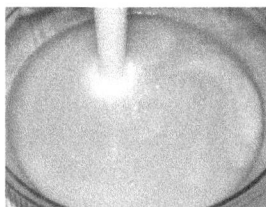

The mass gradually begins to thicken.

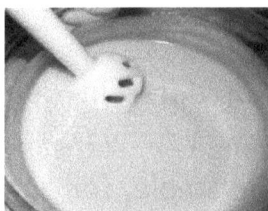

Whisk until the "trace" is visible: when the mass flowing down from the blender, leaves a mark on the surface. Getting the soap mass to the "trace" state generally takes from 5 to 15 minutes to an hour, if you brew soap rich in olive oil. If the blender is overheated stop it every 2 minutes, continue stirring the mass vigorously with a spoon. If the blender is powerful enough, the mass can be brought to trace state without stopping.

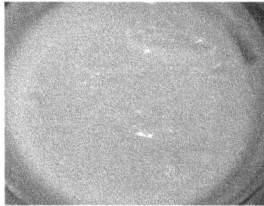

Mass may be of different density, it all depends on how you want to decorate your soap. For example, for a swirl type a very thin faint "footprint'' is needed. Interesting effects can be achieved also with "thick trace".

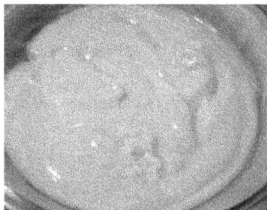

Step 7. Getting to the "trace" state, stop whisking and add dyes, essential oils, useful supplements.

Step 8. Place soap mass into the mold. Wrap the soap in a good towel or a thick cloth and leave to harden about a day. For the soap quickly matures, it must pass the stage of "gel": as a result of chemical reactions soap heats up, it becomes soft and translucent, like a gel. To speed up this process, put it in a warm bur switched off oven. If you make milk soap and want to preserve its whiteness you should, on the contrary, avoid passing the "gel" stage: put soap in a cool place (in the freezer, for example).

Step 9. When the soap hardens (about a day), remove it from the mold and cut into portion pieces. Use gloves, because soaping process has not finished yet and alkali can damage the skin. Cut pieces of soap and leave to dry and ripen in a well ventilated dark place for three to four weeks.

As you can see - it is very easy! The most difficult is to wait until this wonderful piece of homemade soap ripens!

I will conclude with a master class of making soap from scratch by a cold process method.

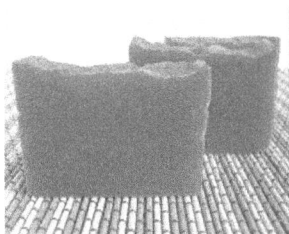

For the preparation of soap you will need:

• sunflower oil - 20 g.

• coconut oil - 120 g.,

• castor oil - 50 g.

• olive oil - 85 g.,

• palm oil - 200 g.,

• alkali (NaOH) - 65,9 g.,

• Water - 156.75 g.,

• Coloring agents and fragrances - any desired.

You will also need:

• gauze,

• scales

• wooden spoon,

• thermometer of 100 degrees,

• blender,

• form (mold) for soap - best of wood: it retains heat well. But do not take glass or metal! Form may be paved from the inside with a paper for the ready soap would be easier to get.

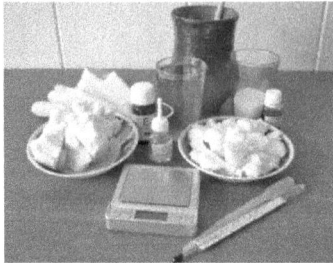

For making soap from scratch by cold pulping method it is better to take non-carbonated mineral water or purified bottled. **Water should be pre-cooled** - it should be very cold!

Workplace Preparation:

1. Cover the table and floor with newspapers or oilcloth to avoid damage if alkaline solution suddenly gets on it.

2. Wear apron (rubber or oilcloth), gloves (rubber or latex).

3. Put nearby a bottle with vinegar to neutralize the alkali, if it suddenly gets on your skin.

4. Wear goggles and a respirator (when you're mixing and adding alkali to a solution). Always keep these rules to protect yourself from harmful alkali vapors!

Step by step preparation of soap from scratch by cold method

1. Take solid oils and melt them over a water bath, stirring occasionally with a spoon.

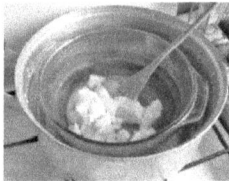

2. Once they meld down completely, pour them into liquid oil.

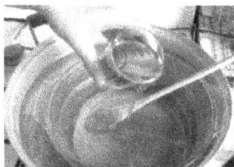

3. Measure the temperature of the oil with thermometer. At the temperature of 60 degrees, remove the oil from the water bath.

4. Take specified quantity of water and alkali. Pour alkali only with a spoon, not over the edge of dishes! Disposable cups may be used when weighing alkali, but working with them it is not very convenient, since they are soft. It is better to allocate for it special glasses, and not use them ever again.

5. Slowly pour the alkali into ice water (not vice versa), stirring the solution. Do this

job on the balcony at the open windows or turning on the conditioner. Do not forget to wear a respirator!

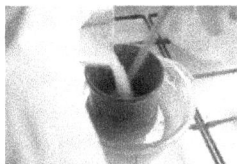

6. When the alkali is completely dissolved, the solution becomes clear. But if not all particles of alkaline solution are dissolved, the solution should be strained through gauze. Then put it in a bag, tie and immediately throw away! Instead of gauze you can't use metal strainers!

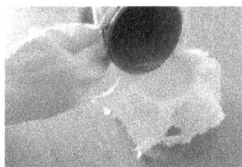

7. Measure the temperature of the oil and alkaline solution. It should be about the

same - 50-55 degrees - the temperature difference should not be more than 1-2 degrees. Now you can start to mix them: pour alkali into oil, stirring slowly.

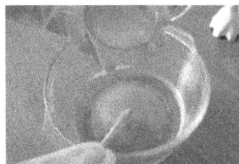

8. Now you can remove protection means (except for gloves) and begin mixing with a blender (not a mixer!) until there is the trace. The "trace" begins to appear on the band when the mass becomes sufficiently dense. The whole process can take from 3 to 10 minutes. But usually 3-4 minutes are enough. If there is no blender, you can mix with a spoon, but it will be quite long.

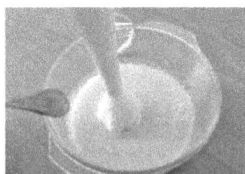

9. Once the "trace" appeared, begin to act very quickly! **The mass almost instantly begins to freeze.** Add colors and flavors and quickly stir everything well.

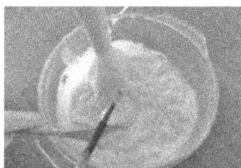

10. Pour the soap into the mold, tamp well with spoon and then tap the shape on the table, so that the ready soap does not have holes.

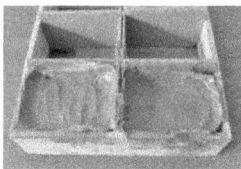

11. Wrap up warmly in some warm cloth and place in a preheated (but powered-off!) to 100 degree oven for **8 hours**. You need to remove soap for a few times during this process, preheat the oven and put it back. You should do this to pass the gel stage. Gel stage looks like this:

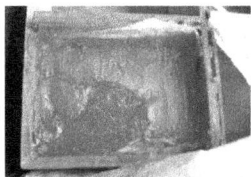

12. After completing the soap gel stage, keep it wrapped up for the rest of **48 hours** in the room temperature. Then remove the soap from the mold. It should be done with gloves - soap can still strongly pinch the skin, causing irritation. Cut it into pieces, wrap each in greaseproof paper, fold in the cloth bag and forget about it **for 2 months**: so long will the soap from scratch ripen. When

time comes, you'll see that you have got a lovely soap that does not dry the skin, cleans well, smells amazing, and most importantly, it is made with your own hands!

Chapter 11: Choosing Equipment

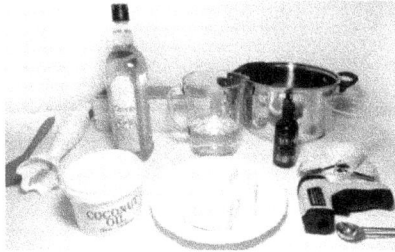

Goggles and rubber gloves

Safety is always first. You cannot skip these essential items of equipment at all. Make sure you wear protective gloves for your hands and protective eye goggles for eye protection to protect against the irritant lye solution and during mixing soap.

Spatulas and spoons for stirring

You will need rubber ones for scraping off the last bits of mix from the soap pot. You will also need wooden ones for stirring.

Plastic could also work but make sure it is heat resistant to resist the heat emitted when the saponification reaction takes place.

A digital scale or a kitchen scale for measuring and measuring cups

Accurate measurement of ingredients is the key to nailing the soap recipe successfully. You need a sensitive scale to accurately measure the weight of lye, distilled water, oils and even dye powder.

Soap pot

You can use stainless steel or plastic large pots. It is better to have large pots so that you mix everything at once, instead of making smaller batches. This is the pot you will use for mixing your soap.

Thermometer

You need to be able to quickly and accurately measure the temperature of oils and the lye water

Mold

The soap making process is not complete without pouring your mixture into a mold. You can purchase a specific soap mold or you can use any house old item that fits the purpose such as an old yoghurt containers or plastic containers.

Stick blender

To start the saponification process and reach the trace, you need a hand blender that will speed up the saponification process. You can stir by hand but that would take hours.

Measuring cups

You will need various containers for measuring up your ingredients before weighing them or for measuring your dye and fragrance.

Glass pitcher

This is for mixing lye; it is preferred to label it "Hazardous" to indicate caution and to ensure people stay away from it. You may need another one to weigh in and heat your oil in.

Additional

You may need professional soap cutters to cut out the bars. You may also need stamps for decorative purposes or for professional labeling.

Soap making ingredients

Soap base

There are several options to choose from when selecting a base. Clear and White Melt and Pour is a good place to start. They're simple, cleansing, and ready to customize. The clear base will have more bright colors, while the white will have more pastel colors. You can also try bases with additives like shea butter, goat milk, or aloe vera.

Melt and pour soapmaking involves melting and customizing pre-made soap bases. Melt and pour soap is quick to make and doesn't need to be cured like cold process soap. As soon as the soap hardens and cools, it's ready to go! Melt and pour soap does not require handling sodium hydroxide lye, making it a fun project for beginners and children. It also lends itself better than cold process soap to certain techniques, like incredibly crisp and clean lines.

If you're thinking about making melt and pour soap, the first step is to choose a base! With so many different options, it can be a little overwhelming. There are a wide variety of bases, each with different ingredients which will affect how they behave, look and feel on the skin. The type of base you use will most likely depend on the design of your project, budget and personal preference.

Melt and pour bases need to be chopped into small pieces before melting. Then the base is ready to customize with color, fragrance and more!

First, it's important to understand how melt and pour soap is different from cold process soap, and how it is similar. Both cold process and melt and pour soap are created by mixing lye and oils to start the saponification process. When these ingredients are measured correctly, there is no lye in the final bar of soap. During the soapmaking process, melt and pour soap has extra glycerin added. Glycerin is a humectant that draws moisture to the skin. The glycerin content in melt and pour soap is also what makes it possible to melt down melt and pour soap to a liquid texture that's easy to work with. It's also the reason that glycerin dew can form on melt and pour soap.

About SFIC Melt and Pour Bases:

SFIC Melt and Pour Bases have the most options to choose from. These bases are also referred to as the "premium" or "house" bases. SFIC is the manufacturer of the bases, and has been producing soap bases since 1967. If you'd like to learn more about SFIC, click here. The ingredients primarily consist of coconut oil, palm oil, safflower oil, glycerin, water and sodium hydroxide. The remaining ingredients depend on the base. For example, the Goat Milk Melt and Pour Base is the only SFIC base that contains goat milk, and the Hemp Melt and Pour Soap Base is the only base that contains hemp seed oil. Can't decide which base is the perfect one for you? The Melt and Pour Sampler Kit includes one pound of the most popular bases.

These bases come in three size options: 1 pound, 10 pounds and 50 pounds. The 1 pound blocks (shown below) come wrapped and labeled. The 10 pound and 50 pound options are shipped unwrapped and come in random size blocks. Because melt and pour is chopped into small pieces before melting, the size of the block doesn't make much difference. If you prefer wrapped, consistent sized blocks, ordering multiple 1 pound blocks is the way to go. =) Some of the more popular bases also come in 25 pound blocks. These include Clear Melt and Pour Base, Goat Milk Melt and Pour Base and White Melt and Pour Base.

All of the SFIC bases are made with high quality ingredients, and do not contain detergents to create lather, such as SLS. Because of the high quality, they are a little bit more expensive than other base options. To compare and contrast the ingredients of these bases, check out the list below!

About Bulk Melt and Pour Bases:

If you are looking for a more cost effective base, the Bramble Berry Bulk Melt and Pour Bases are a great option. Unique to Bramble Berry, you won't find this formula anywhere else. The bulk bases are made with a higher amount of glycerin than the "Premium" bases, and contain SLS (Sodium Lauryl Sulfate). Sodium lauryl sulfate is a synthetic lathering agent that is used to give the bulk bases a creamy lather. These bases feel amazing on the skin, but if you prefer a more "natural" base, the premium SFIC bases may be a better option for you.

The minimum purchase size of Bramble Berry Bulk Bases are 25 pounds. The bases come in 25 pound blocks, which are encased in a plastic bag inside of the box. This is poured directly into the box by the soap maker, so there are usually little bubbles or foam at the top of the block.

About Stephenson Melt and Pour Bases:

The Stephenson melt and pour bases are a new addition to the Bramble Berry product line. These bases are created by Stephenson Personal Care, a company that offers a wide variety of personal care bases including lotion, conditioner and more. You can find all their products here. Bramble Berry currently offers these melt and pour soap bases by Stephenson: African Black Soap Melt and Pour, Goat Milk Melt and Pour, Oatmeal and Shea Melt and Pour, SLS Free Clear Melt and Pour, Jelly Melt and Pour and Suspending Melt and Pour. All of these bases have unique properties that make them distinct options from both the bulk bases, and the premium SFIC bases.

The Jelly Melt and Pour Base has a fun, wiggly texture that makes it completely different from all other melt and pour options. Click here to see it in action in the Shimmery Summer Soap Jellies. The

137

Suspending Melt and Pour Base has a thicker texture than most bases, which makes it perfect for suspending heavier additives like jojoba beads.

Lye

It is sodium hydroxide, an alkali substance used in oven cleaners etc. It is caustic and highly irritant, but it is critical to the saponification process. Lye can result from the white ashes of extremely burnt wood at very high temperatures. It is used in drain cleaners. Don't buy drain cleaners to use for the soap making process. Buy the raw lye. Make sure you buy 100% lye. To ensure a pure product, buy it directly from the manufacturer.

Glycerin

Glycerin is a natural byproduct of the saponification process. It's one of the reasons handmade soap feels so amazing – it draws moisture to the skin and keeps it hydrated. Additional glycerin is added during the melt and pour manufacturing process to make it easy to work with. It can also cause the soap to sweat in humid climates, so make sure to wrap your bars and keep them in a cool, dry place.

Are there beads of liquid on your melt and pour soap, or do the bars look powdery? Are they slippery and wet to the touch? This is a common reaction referred to as "sweating" or "glycerin dew."

Melt and pour soap has extra glycerin added during the manufacturing process. It makes the soap easy to work with and also acts as a humectant. When you wash with melt and pour soap, a thin layer of glycerin is left behind. That draws moisture from the air onto your skin. Learn more about what the bases are made with in this Sunday Night Spotlight.

As melt and pour soap sits on the counter, glycerin draws moisture onto the bars and forms glycerin dew. It's more common in humid climates.

The good news is that it's easy to prevent with the following tips.

The Like Cold Process (LCP) Clear and LCP White bases have less glycerin, which means there's little to no sweating. They're a good option for extremely humid climates. We also recommend the LCP bases if you're embedding melt and pour in cold process soap because they don't morph or sweat as the bars cure.

Let the soap harden and cool at room temperature. If it's placed in the fridge or freezer for long periods of time it's more likely to sweat.

Wrap the bars tightly with plastic wrap and use a heat gun to shrink it on tightly. This Soap Queen TV video shows you how.

Run a fan over the soap once it's out of the mold. This is a good option for moderately humid climates but likely won't work for extremely humid climates.

Buy a dehumidifier and use it in your soaping space. It's a good investment because it creates a dry environment for other products like cold process soap and bath bombs.

You can also place the wrapped bars in an airtight container with rice or silica packets. Learn more in How to Store Handmade Bath Products.

Molds

You need to use a mold that can withstand higher temperatures so it doesn't melt when you pour in hot soap. You also want it to be flexible so it's easy to unmold the bars.

Oils

The type of oil affects the hardness and lather of the soap. The combination of oils you chose for the soap can be optimized to achieve the hardness or softness you want.

Coconut Oil - Hard, lots of lather, makes the soap drying. Add more fat to soften the soap, although it gives good consistency.

Palm Oil - Hard, makes a long-lasting bar. Mild lather. Great alternative to animal fat.

Olive oil - Soft, low cleansing effects, and offers a slippery lather. Castile soap is 100% olive oil. It is suitable for sensitive skin. Takes a longer time to cure and harden. It is better to use extra virgin oil.

Lard - Hard, has a creamy lather. 100% lard can be a great laundry soap.

Cocoa butter - brittle and long-lasting bar. Creamy lather.

Shea Butter - Hard, medium creamy lather, long-lasting bar.

Castor oil - Improves the lather by improving soap solubility.

Other options - Avocado oil, almond oil, palm kernel oil.

Fragrances and essential oils

You can scent your soap with fragrance oils or essential oils. A general usage rate is about 0.3 oz. of scent per pound of soap. Find light, medium, and strong recommendations with the Fragrance Calculator. It's important to use skin-safe scents like the ones from Bramble Berry. Potpourri, craft, or candle fragrances may not be skin safe or tested in soap. Be sure to check with the manufacturer before use.

Fragrance oil is a mixture of natural and synthetic, carefully blended after lots of trials to provide an alluring and captivating scent. Many of them are thinned and diluted to have the perfume/scent quality. There are safe soap fragrance oils that are safe to your skin but make sure it is designed for soap to ensure its safety.

Essential oils are natural and made from plants by capturing the essence of the plant. The oil can be taken from various parts of the plant, depending on the plant. It can be seeds or leaves. Fragrances and essential oils are a wonderful addition to your product. Experiment with different oils. Some recipes guide you which oils to use. You can use either or a mix of both.

Herbs, roots, flowers, petals, fruits

Some recipes make use of herbs such as tea, lavender or even coffee beans. Keep your mind open to new variations. You can dice up fruit such as pumpkins or grate cucumber peel to add a beautiful touch.

Colorants

It is a wonderful addition to add color to your soap. There are plenty of options for coloring melt and pour soap. Micas and color blocks are easy to use and they look great in the finished bars. Learn more about how to work with our skin-safe soap colorants in this post. We don't recommend options like food coloring or crayons because they haven't been tested or approved for use in soap. They tend to morph, fade, or bleed. Lavender smelling soap could be colored purple to compliment the mental image. Some recipes offer natural coloring like cucumber infused recipes.

Decorating your soap

You can get very creative with your soap, starting with picking the shape of the mold or creating your own mold. Another great method would be to swirl the soap or use certain dividers in a way that creates new designs. The malleability of soap allows you to make it into any shape you desire easily. You can even cut the soap into small heart shaped pieces and put them in a jar with a cute note or shape it as cookies or anything you literally want.

Coloring is another great thing to get creative with when designing. You can create master pieces and color combinations. It is a great idea to have inspiration on how to design your soap.

You can also use the edge of the spoon to engrave patterns in the soap, insert petals, rhinestones, glitter, herbs, secret message inside. Literally anything you want. Certain petals can add a luxurious touch to your soap. It is really up to your creativity. You can also buy a stamp that makes cute shapes on the surface of the soap or engraves your trademark.

The packaging of the soap itself is an important factor in how professional and appealing your soap looks. Make sure the soap edges are cut neatly and smoothly as well as evenly. Invest in some creative and cute packing, make it personal and make it lovely.

Chapter 12: 20 Nourishing Cold Process Soap Recipes

Now it's your turn to make some soap! Use the cold-process soap making process you just learned about to make the below recipes – and remember, have fun!

All recipes will produce 5 pounds of soap. All weights are in ounces (by weight, not by volume unless for additives).

Simply Soothing Soap

This is a no frills, uncomplicated recipe that you can tweak with different essential oils and colorants. One of the hardest parts of cold process soap making is recognizing trace. Test for trace frequently to make sure you don't miss it! If you keep stirring for too long, your soap will likely solidify in the pot. 26.5 ounces olive oil

16.5 ounces coconut oil

10 ounces palm oil

7.37 ounces lye

20 ounces distilled water

Temperature to adjust to ("wait and adjust"): 95 degrees

Insulation time: one full day

Curing time: 4-6 weeks

Luxurious Lavender Soap

This soap, which includes oats and lavender, is soothing for skin and helps provide an aromatherapy experience. This recipe is also 5% superfatted!

21.2 ounces olive oil

10.6 ounces palm oil

3.18 ounces shea butter

4.77 ounces rice bran oil

10.6 ounces coconut oil

2.65 ounces castor oil

2.65 ounces lavender oil

4 tablespoons colloidal oatmeal (finely ground whole oats)

20 ounces oat milk* (instead of water)

7.27 grams lye

Optional: lavender buds for decoration after pouring into molds

*How to make oat milk:

Mix one cup of whole oats (not quick oats) with three cups of water and blend on high until smooth. Strain over cheesecloth or a fine strainer.

Temperature to adjust to ("wait and adjust"): 110 degrees

Insulation time: one full day

Curing time: 6-8 weeks

Honey Oatmeal Soap

This soap smells delicious and includes therapeutic clove bud and sweet orange essential oils. You'll want to add your almond milk immediately after you pour the lye into your oils mixture so the mix doesn't get too thick. Stir manually for a few minutes, then go ahead and add the honey, then the oatmeal, then the essential oils.

26.5 ounces olive oil

10.6 ounces coconut oil

6.4 ounces sweet almond oil

5.3 ounces avocado oil

4.3 ounces castor oil

2.5 ounces honey diluted with 3 ounces of warm water

6 ounces almond milk

2 ounces whole oats (to sprinkle on top after pouring into mold)

1.59 ounces sweet orange essential oil

1.06 ounces clove bud essential oil

12 ounces water

7.28 ounces lye

Temperature to adjust to ("wait and adjust"): 80-90 degrees

Insulation time: one full day

Curing time: 6-8 weeks

Cup Of Coffee Soap

This bar of soap won't wake you up in the morning quite as well as a cup of coffee, but its delicious aroma will make for the perfect morning shower. Do not add powdered cinnamon or nutmeg instead of essential oils to your mixture as they can irritate the skin!

23.85 ounces olive oil

8.5 ounces coconut oil

10.6 ounces palm oil

5.3 ounces rice bran oil

2.65 ounces sweet almond oil

2.1 ounces castor oil

1.34 ounces coffee essential oil

.332 ounces nutmeg essential oil

6 ounces strong brewed coffee, cooled (to be added with the essential oils in the "customize" step)

14 ounces water

7.2 ounces lye

Temperature to adjust to ("wait and adjust"): 90-100 degrees

Insulation time: 12-24 hours

Curing time: 6-8 weeks

Smooth As Silk Shaving Bar

You'll love the rich lather and protective layer this shaving bar will provide. Use with a shaving brush for luxurious results. Mix the bentonite clay in very slowly to prevent clumping. Add the bentonite clay first, then the oatmeal.

23.9 ounces olive oil

10.6 ounces coconut oil

10.6 ounces castor oil

4.2 ounces palm oil

3.7 ounces sweet almond oil

3 tablespoons bentonite clay

4 tablespoons colloidal oatmeal

20 ounces water

7.27 ounces lye

Temperature to adjust to ("wait and adjust"): 110 degrees

Insulation time: Do not insulate your soap to allow it to stay very creamy. Let it solidify for 12-24 hours.

Curing time: 4-6 weeks

2-Pound Batch Cold Process Soap Recipes

For readers who may not want to make as much as 5-pound batches, the following recipes are about 2 pounds each. These are perfect for a 10-inch loaf mold, making about 7-8 4-ounce bars. For cold process soaps, you will want your oils and lye mixture to cool to about 100-120F before mixing. Soaps should be insulated for 24-48 hours, and cure for 3-4 weeks before use (exclusive of Castile soap).

Pomegranate Exfoliation Bar

The super fruit pomegranate is also great for your skin, offering moisturizing, anti-oxidant, and anti-inflammatory properties. This simple recipe gives you extra exfoliating power with pomegranate powder.

7 ounces coconut oil

7 ounces olive oil

7 ounces vegetable shortening

3 ounces lye

6.8 ounces distilled water

1.6 ounces pomegranate fragrance oil

2 tbsp. pomegranate powder

red dye colorant

Add the pomegranate powder in the "Customize" step.

Ginger Lime Soap

The zing of sparkling ginger and fresh lime makes this bar the perfect morning pick-me-up soap. This recipe employs just an ounce of beeswax for additional hardness, ensuring that the bar will last longer.

1 ounce sweet almond oil

4 ounces canola oil

3 ounces castor oil

8 ounces coconut oil

3 ounces olive oil

3 ounces palm oil

1 ounce beeswax

7 ounces distilled water

3.24 ounces lye

1.4 ounce ginger lime fragrance oil

Yellow and green pigment-type colorant

In the "Customize" step, after adding your fragrance oil, divide the batch between two bowls, adding green colorant to one and yellow to the other. Pour the green into molds first and give it a minute or two to harden; then add the yellow to give your soap a layered look.

Bringin' Home The Bacon Lard Soap

Reminiscent of soaps of yore, this simple bar relies solely on lard for the fat content. Contrary to what some may believe, lard doesn't make soap greasy but is, in fact, mild, moisturizing and conditioning. For this novelty soap, I use bacon fragrance oil to really go whole hog.

22 ounces lard

8 ounces distilled water

2.84 ounces lye

1.2 ounces bacon fragrance oil

Mango Papaya Soap

This fruity soap smells good enough to eat! With an addition of castor oil and shea butter, this bar is both bubbly and silky. For this recipe I like to give the soap a pretty marbled effect using vibrant mica powder.

4 ounces castor oil

5 ounces coconut oil

5 ounces olive oil

3 ounces palm oil

3 ounces shea butter

2 ounces sweet almond oil

8 ounces distilled water

3 ounces lye

1.6 ounces mango papaya fragrance oil

½ tablespoon red-orange mica powder

In the "Customize" step, after adding your fragrance oil, divide the batch between two bowls. Blend the mica powder into one bowl. Pour the un-colored soap into your mold(s), followed by the red-orange soap. Using a skewer or butter knife, gently cut paths through the soap to swirl the colors, giving a beautiful marbled effect.

Lemongrass Green Tea Soap

Green tea is known to help prevent skin aging and has natural anti-inflammatory properties. Not only does this soap have a soothing scent, it employs dried lemongrass to gently exfoliate as you wash. If you can't find green tea butter, substitute with sweet almond oil.

2 ounces castor oil

8 ounces coconut oil

2 ounces green tea butter

4 ounces olive oil

16 ounces vegetable shortening

10 ounces strong brewed green tea

4.43 ounces lye

1.5 ounce lemongrass & green tea fragrance oil

.25 ounces lemongrass essential oil

2-4 tablespoons dried lemongrass

Stir in the dried lemongrass in the "Customize" stage. Save a little bit to sprinkle over your soap after you pour it into the mold(s).

Honey Apricot Soap

When used in just small amounts honey can greatly increase the benefits of your soap. Aside from giving your bar a nice moisturizing lather, it also has antimicrobial and anti-inflammatory properties that cleanse and soothe the skin.

4.4 ounces canola oil

5.5 ounces coconut oil

2.2 ounces jojoba oil

4.4 ounces olive oil

5.5 ounces palm oil

2 tbsp. honey

1.6 ounces honeyed apricot fragrance oil

Add the honey in the "Customize" step.

Goat's Milk & Honey Soap

Goat's milk has become a popular soap making base- and for a good reason. It contains alpha hydroxy acids that get rid of dead skin cells, a number of vitamins and minerals, moisturizing cream, and anti-bacterial properties. This bar is great for people with acne or other skin conditions.

1 ounce castor oil

5 ounces coconut oil

4.25 ounces olive oil

11 ounces vegetable shortening

3 ounces lye

12 ounces frozen, partially thawed goat milk

1.2 ounces Goat's Milk & Honey fragrance oil

2 tbsp. honey

Be sure to work slowly when adding lye to milk as it can scald easily and discolor your soap.

100% Castile

Castile soap gets its name from the Castile region of Spain, where bars of this hard olive-based soap have been made for hundreds of years. Bergamont essential oil adds a uplifting, mood enhancing appeal to this 100% olive oil soap. Be warned, this soap takes a lot of patience. For the best possible bar, you must wait at least 4 months for the soap to cure.

22 ounces olive oil

8 ounces distilled water

2.8 ounces lye

1.4 ounces bergamont essential oil

Nuts About Almond Soap

This soap recipe features almond, almond, and more almond in the form of oil, butter, and milk. I've also added a yummy almond fragrance oil to really make that warm, nutty scent pop. As opposed to a water base, the use of almond milk in this recipe adds extra skin nourishing benefits, but feel free to use water if you can't find any.

3 ounces almond butter

2 ounces sweet almond oil

2 ounces castor oil

6 ounces coconut oil

5 ounces olive oil

6 ounces vegetable shortening

6 ounces almond milk

3.3 ounces lye

1.4 ounces almond fragrance oil

Monkey Farts Soap For Kids

Don't let the name fool you, this combination of tropical fruits, banana and creamy coconut smells divine, and is especially popular with kids...or kids of all ages. The extra castor oil gives the soap a nice bubbly later, and the funky color blend makes this a soap that the young ones will love.

2.2 ounces canola oil

1.3 ounces castor oil

5.5 ounces coconut oil

5.5 ounces olive oil

5.5 ounces palm oil

2.2 ounces sunflower seed oil

7.3 ounces distilled water

3.1 ounces lye

1.7 ounces Monkey Farts fragrance oil

1 tsp. each hot pink, blue, and yellow oxide colorants

Before you begin, mix 1 tsp. of colorant with 1 tbsp. of olive oil in three separate bowls using a whisk or mini mixer. At trace, separate your soap into three bowls and add one mixed color to each. When you pour the soap into your molds, alternate colors and swirl.

Coconut Salt Scrub Bar

This tropical treat uses sea salt to gently exfoliate as you wash. Since the fats are 80% coconut oil it makes a nice hard bar. This soap is 50% salt, so it must be cut before completely set to avoid crumbling.

1.2 ounces avocado oil

2 ounces castor oil

12.8 ounces coconut oil

5.3 ounces coconut milk

2.4 ounces lye

16 ounces medium grain sea salt

1.6 ounces coconut fragrance oil

Before you begin, preheat the oven to 170F. Add the sea salt in the "Customize" step, and stir well before pouring into your mold. Place the mold in the heated oven and turn off the heat. Allow the soap to sit for about 2 hours until it is firm.

Immediately cut into bars and set aside to cure.

Salted Caramel

Salted caramel is all the rage these days. Now you can rub the delicious aroma all over your skin! A small amount of fine sea salt adds to the longevity and cleansing power of the bar.

2 ounces castor oil

12 ounces coconut oil

4 ounces olive oil

2 ounces shea butter

2.89 ounces lye

6.6 ounces milk of your choice (cow, goat, almond, rice, whatever you have on hand!)

1.5 ounces caramel or salted caramel fragrance oil

7 ounces fine grain sea salt, 1 tbsp. reserved for topping

1 tsp. bronze mica powder

Add the salt and mica powder in the "Customize" step, blending thoroughly. After pouring into your mold, top with reserved salt.

The Bee's Knees Honeysuckle Soap

A little bit of beeswax goes a long way to contribute to the hardness of this bar. This floral soap will make you think of springtime, when the honeysuckle is just beginning to bloom. Place bubble wrap on top of your freshly poured soap to give it a neat honeycomb effect.

.42 ounces beeswax

1 ounce castor oil

5.9 ounces coconut oil

5.9 ounces olive oil

5.9 ounces palm oil

2.59 ounces lye

7 ounces water

1.3 ounces honeysuckle fragrance oil

2 tablespoons honey

Add honey in the "Customize" step.

Homemade Shampoo Bar

Homemade soap isn't just for your skin! This nifty shampoo bar uses castor and coconut oils for a nice bubbly lather, while sweet almond and jojoba oils help to condition your hair.

2.1 ounces canola oil

4.2 ounces castor oil

5.25 ounces coconut oil

1 ounce jojoba oil

4.2 ounces olive oil

2.1 ounces palm oil

2.1 ounces sweet almond oil

2.85 ounces lye

6.9 ounces water

1.5 ounces fragrance oil of choice- crisp apple, tropical coconut, and citrus splash are great options

Chocolate Lovers Soap

This delectable recipe triples up on the chocolate with cocoa butter for firmness and moisturizing qualities, cocoa powder for color, and chocolate fragrance oil for a strong, lasting scent. A chocoholic's dream!

2.2 ounces castor oil

2.2 ounces cocoa butter, non-deodorized

6.6 ounces coconut oil

6.6 ounces olive oil

4.4 ounces palm oil

3 ounces lye

7.26 ounces water

1.5 ounces chocolate fragrance oil

1 tbsp. cocoa powder

Add the cocoa powder in the "Customize" step.

Chapter 13: Basic Soap Recipes

Learning basic recipes is very important if you want to start customizing your soap. Here are some of the most common basic soap recipes that you can later on in the next chapter learn how to incorporate fragrances, colorants, and herbs in.

The following recipes use the cold process method. The steps are in basic format and can be used the same in each recipe.

Here's a quick guide to the cold process method if needed while following the sample recipes. (The more detailed version can be found in the previous chapter)

Step 1 Prepare. **Mix the lye solution then set aside.** Measure carefully and heat your solid oils until their completely melted. Then measure and add the liquid oils to the melted solid oils.

173

Step 2 **Combine.** When the lye and the oils are at about 100-110 degrees, very slowly pour the lye solution into the oils. Stir mixture with a stick blender, making sure to alternate short blasts with the blender and stirring.

Step 3 **Stirring**. Keep mixing the soap until it reaches a light trace.

Step 4 **Fragrance.** Add the fragrance oil. Mix them into the soap thoroughly.

Step 5 **Mold.** Ready your mold then carefully pour the raw soap mixture in. Then let it cool for 12-24 hours or until it's hard enough to cut.

Step 6 **Cure.** Let it cure for 2-4 weeks.

The 4-oil soap bar

6.5 oz. Coconut oil

6.5 oz. Palm oil

7.5 oz. Olive oil

1.3 oz. Castor oil

8 oz. Water

3.1oz. Lye

1 oz. Of fragrance oil or essential oil

Lavender Bar

4.23 oz Water

2.25 oz. lye

3.9 oz coconut oil

5.78 oz. olive oil

2.9 oz. palm oil

2.75 sun flower oil

0.67 oz she butter

0.4 oz lavender essential oil

Violent colorant (optional)

Lavender buds (optional

** Add essential oil and lavender buds once the trace is notices,

Honey And Oats Bar

4.23 oz. water

2.22 oz. lye

4.8 oz. coconut oil

6.9 oz. olive oil

2.4 oz. castor oil

1.6 oz. palm oil

0.32 oz. bee's wax

0.25 oz. honey

0.07 oz. rolled oats

**Add honey once trace is noticed and whisk well. Then add oats.

Making It your Own

The sky is the limit when creating your own soap recipes but remember, it all boils down to basic chemistry. Your process should stay at the basic until you're comfortable enough to experiment. Here are some tips on brainstorming your soap creations.

Who's the soap for?

Make your soap to fit your market's needs. Are you making it for a friend or family member? Or maybe you want to use it as a display piece for your guest room? If it's for an aspiring business then you've got a lot of planning to do. There's much to consider. The herbs and oils you use may irritate the skin of someone who is hyper sensitive or allergic. If your market is Vegan you'll have to cut out all animal products like lard, honey and beeswax.

Where you're located can play a big factor in the type of ingredients that are available to you.

Before anything, do your research on the type of soap you want to make and who it's for.

All about oils

Every bar of soap needs oil or fat and the type you use can change the bar completely. Here's a list of how common oil affects the results of your bar.

Cleansing oils: Coconut oil, sunflower oil

For extra lather: Canola oil, coco butter, hempseed oil, jojoba

Conditioning oil: avocado oil, Mango butter, grape seed oil, olive oil, Shea butter, almond oil, corn oil

For a hard bar: beeswax, lanolin, lard, palm oil, tallow

Essential Oils

Essential oils are a natural oil concentration from flowers, fruits and herbs which can give your soap lasting benefits.

The type of essential oil you use is entirely up to you. The rule of thumb when adding essential oils to your recipe is never exceed %3 of your total recipe. Doing so will overpower your soap in a bad way.

Dressing it up

Now that you've successfully made the soap of dreams, it's time to dress it up. Normally, people will be attracted to the look and smell of your soap before making a purchase so packaging is vital when before selling. The possibilities are endless when it comes to the material and technique available. No worries, here's a thorough list of creative packaging ideas.

For wrapping:

Cellophane may be the cheapest form of wrapping soap and it keeps fragrance locked in but also prevents shoppers from getting a sniff of your product. Some soap makers just punch several tiny holes in the cellophane to release some aroma. Good for all shapes and sizes of soap.

Printed paper is a smart approach because it's a 2-in-1 wrapper and label. The printed paper can be used to wrap the entire bar of soap or with cigar style method which will be explained in the next section. This styling method is for the clean and simple soap maker.

The box with window style is a pricier option but does two useful things at once. It keeps the soap in good condition by protecting it and it allows the shopper to sniff, see and feel the soap through the window.

Holiday gift baskets and boxes are a wonderful investment for soap makers who are serious about their profit. Gift baskets can be lined with wrapping tissues, straw, or confetti. Also, make sure to make your Logo easy to catch. You never know who your basket is going to. Use your imagination when creating these because the more creative and cared for these gift baskets are, the more you will sell!

Decorative wrapping tissues come in many variations. Some of them are made from recycled or natural materials. Others are very fine and delicate for the high end soap makers. Wrapping tissues can be directly wrapped on the soap or used as a lining for soap boxes or bags as mentioned earlier.

Paper bags are a great idea for soap samples as you can put a variation of small soaps in it without spending too much. Use a cutter to place a heart-shaped hole on the top for a visual appeal. You might even want to slide a business card inside.

Shrink wrapping is ideal for a soap maker who wants to keep the soap well-preserved. When soap is left uncovered it allows water to evaporate prolonging the curing process. This is why you sometimes see soap that looks dry or shriveled up.

The half box is the one of the best ways to wrap. It's less expensive than a regular box and leaves one side exposed allowing the aromas out without causing shrinking from prolonged curing.

See through fabric bags are easy and prettier if you're going for a girly look. If you've molded your soap into a unique shape like a leaf or shell it will be easier to package and see. They may also attract buyers because they can be re-used after the soap is gone.

Scrubby bags are a favorite but quite pricey. It's basically a small bag made out of exfoliating fabric. The soap stays inside so all you have to do is add water and lather for maximum scrubbing!

Coffee Filter/Round papers are normally used for round soap as they're a better fit. Of course round papers can be more expensive than coffee filters but are versatile in color and texture.

For labeling and add-ons:

Cigar bands have become a common way for label because you can do so much with them and they're overall affordable. The labels are easy to make and you can use different types of cutters and stamps to decorate them. A lot of soap makers like to simply put the cigar band directly on a bare bar of soap but that often causes shrinkage if the bar isn't use soon.

Medallions are a very cute addition to a cigar band or string (basically anything that wraps around the soap). Some are made or plastic metal or wax.

Ribbon, string and yarn add a wholesome appeal to your soap. It may also make the shopper feel like their opening a gift or a treat for themselves. These are usually placed on top of a paper wrap or cigar band.

Carving your soap takes a certain amount of technique and skill. You'll have to invest in a few carving tools if you want it to look professional. Some soap makers carve flowers, herbs or even their company name directly on their soap.

Listing ingredients

There's a lot of discussion on whether or not listing the ingredients on soap labels is necessary. You may come across shopper's who would prefer to know what the soap is made of, or at least what the basic ingredients are. Especially, the shopper's with allergies or sensitive skin. In the end it's a judgment call.

Chapter 14: Cleaning Up

Now that your soap is made, it is time to clean up. Hopefully you worked in an organized fashion and there were no spills making the cleanup process much easier. When cleaning, remember that lye is now in several places, 2 pots and any tools that you used for mixing. It could also be on your gloves, the thermometer and the scale. It is still unsafe and caustic because it did not have to opportunity to react with a fat and saponify. Raw soap is caustic so be careful while cleaning up. The first step is to deal with the leftover raw soap. Use a rubber spatula to scrape the soap out of your pot and into your molds, the less soap you have in your pot the easier it will be to clean. Now rinse all of your containers and tools. Wipe your pot out with paper towels and dispose of them immediately. It is also possible to use "shop" towels, just leave them out overnight before putting them in the wash so the saponification process from the leftover ingredients will complete and no chemical reactions will occur in the washing machine. Alternatively, you can use a lot of hot water and "real" soap to wash the pot. You could also put all of your tools needing cleaning into the pot, cover it with a lid, and leave it overnight. By the next morning the oils and lye that had remained will be soap. Just clean it up in the sink and dry. Do not wash your materials in your dishwasher; the reaction will cause water to spill out onto your floor.

Storing Soap

After your soap has cured, an appropriate way to store it must be found. Keep in mind that the shelf life of homemade soap is much less than commercially made soap and becomes even shorter if it is not stored properly. Homemade soap can last about a year when kept in a cool, dry spot.

Placing it in an airtight container that is placed in a dark, dry, cool spot is ideal. Once you begin to use your soap, it is important to keep it as dry is possible so that it lasts longer.

Conclusion

Thank you again for downloading this book!

I hope that you have learned a lot about the process of making your own soaps and that you are inspired to take what you have learned and use it as soon as you possibly can.

I am sure that you will love the creative art of soap crafting as much as I do and that you will have many years of fun crafting ahead of you.

Personally, I am always amazed at how much the craft keeps evolving and so I find that I am never bored - my gosh, I still remember a time when I had to get the soap to trace by hand - believe me I am so glad that someone figured out that you could use an immersion blender instead!

Thank you and good luck!ss

www.ingramcontent.com/pod-product-compliance
Lightning Source LLC
Chambersburg PA
CBHW060325030426
42336CB00011B/1205